"We're Not an Ideology But Persons With Human Dignity"

Gender and the Catholic Church, Volume 3

Vivencio Ballano

Published by Vivencio Ballano, 2024.

"WE'RE NOT AN IDEOLOGY BUT PERSONS WITH HUMAN DIGNITY"

First edition. November 2, 2024.

ISBN: 979-8227923479

Written by Vivencio Ballano.

Also by Vivencio Ballano

Gender and the Catholic Church
Why Can't Pope Francis and the Catholic Church Fully Accept the LGBTQI?:
A Sociological-Synodal Exploration and Solution
"We are God's Children Too!": Resisting Homophobia and Natural Law for Full
LGBTQI Integration in the Catholic Church
"We're Not an Ideology But Persons With Human Dignity"
Is Gender the Greatest Threat to Humanity and the Family?: A Sociological
Unmasking of a Moral Panic

My Religious Vocation and Journey Vol. 1
God's Call: Why I Entered the Seminary

Table of Contents

Dedicated to All members of the LGBTQI Community!

"We're not an Ideology but Persons with Human Dignity"

Sociology, Catholic Church's Gender Ideology, and LGBTQI Inclusivity

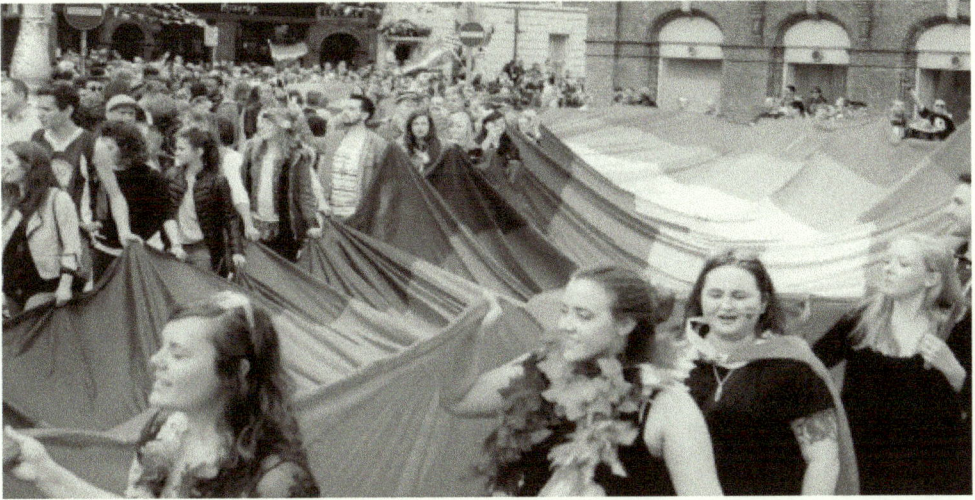

Photo: Dublin LGBTQI Parade **Credit:** Free-Images.com

(Gender and the Catholic Church, #3)

Vivencio O. Ballano

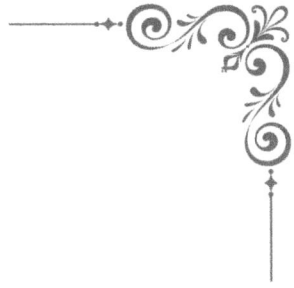

Chapter 1

Book's Overview

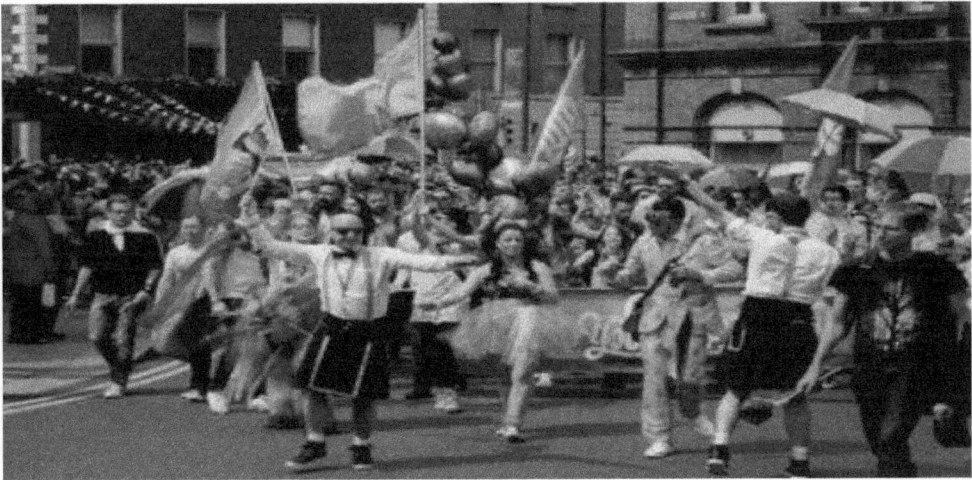

Photo: Dublin LGBTQ Parade **Credit:** Free-Images.com

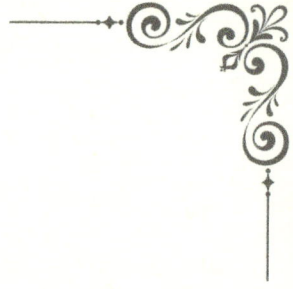

Introduction

I must admit that I was a homophobe or a person with fear of homosexuality and homosexuals before I started doing sociological research and publications on gender and gender diversity. Like any other Catholic heterosexuals as well as Catholic popes such as Pope Benedict XVI, I thought homosexuality is a naturally disordered gender and a deviation of human sexuality.

But after I have read several scientific sociological research and literature as well as online stories about the social discrimination and harassment of non-heterosexuals or members of the so-called lesbian, gay, bisexual, transgender, queer, and intersexual (LGBTQI[1]) community, I gradually became an avid advocate of gender diversity, gender equality, and full LGBTQI inclusion in the Roman Catholic Church and other Christian churches. One of the most painful and touching accounts that I read online on how transgenders and members of the LGBTQI are socially harassed and discriminated both in the church and society is the sad story of a young transgender named Leelah Alcorn, an Ohio teenager, who stepped in front of an oncoming tractor trailer to take her own life.

In her letter posted on Tumblr, Leelah explained why she ended her own life after years of social discrimination and rejection in her school and church because of her transgender identity that her strict Christian parents refused to understand:

> After a summer of having almost no friends plus the weight of having to think about college, save money for moving out, keep my grades up, go to church each week and feel like shit because everyone there is against everything I live for, I have decided I've had enough. I'm never

going to transition successfully, even when I move out. I'm never going to be happy with the way I look or sound. I'm never going to have enough friends to satisfy me. I'm never going to have enough love to satisfy me. I'm never going to find a man who loves me. I'm never going to be happy. Either I live the rest of my life as a lonely man who wishes he were a woman, or I live my life as a lonelier woman who hates herself. There's no winning. There's no way out. I'm sad enough already, I don't need my life to get any worse. People say "it gets better" but that isn't true in my case. It gets worse. Each day I get worse. (Ford Jr.2018, 70).

Leelah further mentioned in her suicide note that she could only rest in peace and make her death memorable if transgenders are treated in society with respect as humans with human rights:

The only way I will rest in peace is if one day transgender people aren't treated the way I was.... [They should be] treated like humans, with valid feelings and human rights[1]. Gender needs to be taught about in schools, the earlier the better. My death needs to mean something. (ABC News 2014, para. 13)

Another teenager named Hope Verbeeck also shared her difficult life living in the closet as a transgender in a suicide note to her parents:

Dear Mommy and Papa, I am so sorry to do this to you, but I have killed myself by jumping off the top floor ... I could no longer live my life as a lie. I'm so sorry I lied to you. I was losing hope in the world and could not see my way out of the wrong body, so I decided it was time for my life to end. Please forgive me for any sins I committed. (Fairchild 2018, para. 23)

Jean-Marie Navetta[2], the Director of Learning & Inclusion for PFLAG, testified about social barriers, discrimination, and harassment encountered by

1. http://abcnews.go.com/topics/news/issues/human-rights.htm
2. https://outreach.faith/
news-views/?_authors=cap-jean-marie-navetta&authors-nn=Jean-Marie%20Navetta

the LGBTQI persons both in society and in their churches such as the Catholic Church:

> I have always considered my life to be blessed. This isn't to say that there haven't been challenges. My life is much like that of any LGBTQ person: barriers exist wherever we go. Even in 2022, when we're more visible than ever, our community lacks basic protections from discrimination in more than half of the United States[3].
>
> And while acceptance has increased in many ways, the attacks on people like me have escalated, too. Sadly, these attacks come often in the name of Jesus Christ.
>
> But when I say my life is blessed, I mean this: Unlike so many people I know in the LGBTQ community, the idea that God loves me less—or not at all—because I happen to be queer has never crossed my mind.
>
> In no uncertain terms, this is a blessing. Stories of alienation from the faith communities in which many of us were raised are painfully common. Worse, too many of us have experienced the weaponization of our religion so often that there's a term for it: spiritual violence.
>
> I know that I'm an exception to the rule. While roughly half of LGBTQI people identify as people of faith (with about 1.3 million identifying as Roman Catholic[4]), a significant portion of us do not participate in the faith communities in which we were raised. (Navetta[5] 2022, paras. 1-5)

In my reflection, I just can't imagine why gays and transgenders should be rejected in the Church and society and be faulted for their non-heterosexual gender and sexuality when, in fact, acquiring one's gender since birth is culturally acquired by the person through the process called gender socialization and or

---

3. https://freedomforallamericans.org/states/

4. https://www.newwaysministry.org/2020/12/11/new-study-nearly-half-of-lgbtq-adults-in-u-s-are-religious-including-many-catholics/

5. https://outreach.faith/news-views/?_authors=cap-jean-marie-navetta&authors-nn=Jean-Marie%20Navetta

social upbringing. I am saddened as a Catholic by the fact that the Catholic Church, which LGBTQI Catholics consider as their spiritual home, would morally judge them as psychological immature and a deviation of human sexuality, and reject them in the Christian community as normal human beings with infinite dignity as Children of God.

The Catholic Church considers "gender" as modern invention of the LGBTQI movement and feminism rather an authentic human experience acquired by the person from the social environment and culture. As one transgender confessed that her nonbinary gender was influenced by her social environment:

> Ever since I was young, I have done life the hard way. This was the same for "coming out". For my whole life I've known that I would be different. In kindergarten I would always play with the girls and sometimes the guys as well, this continued into primary school where I would hang out with the girls, and I was the only boy in the choir. As I went through primary school I started feeling attracted to boys in my class. It wasn't until Year 6 that I started to notice 'being gay', but that just blew over and I thought it was just puberty starting.[2]

Another gay shared her experience how she became a lesbian through social interaction in school:

> From an early age I knew there was something different about me. In primary school I was too young to know I was attracted to the same sex, but I was aware that I behaved differently to the other boys in school. I had some of the typical cliché characteristics of other gay friends of mine growing up. I wasn't interested or good at sports, I was a bit more sensitive and emotionally in tune, and I never understood why it wasn't ok to play with the girls as well as other boys. Nature or nurture I will never know, but most of my gay mates were similar. Not all of us were 'feminine' but most had an awareness that they did not quite fit in.[3]

After reading such stories of social discrimination of the LGBTQI people even in the Catholic Church, I began to wonder why the Church cannot fully accept homosexuals and nonbinary believers in the Christian community. Why can't Catholic bishops and moral theologians see gender as socially learned rather than metaphysically determined? Thus, I began to search for answers. I became curious why the Catholic Church, which is preaching Christ's gospel of love and preferential option for those who are poor, downtrodden, and harassed in society, could fully integrate LGBTQI Catholics with their unique non-heterosexual gender identity. What's wrong with the current moral framework of the Catholic Church that it cannot completely welcome nonbinary believers such as the LGBTQI as Children of God?

Pope Francis is the first Catholic pope to show great compassion for the LGBTQI community in the Catholic Church. He surprised conservative critics when he welcomed Yayo Grassi, his former gay student, and his male partner for 19 years, Iwan Bagus, to a private audience at the Apostolic Nunciature in Washington, D.C., on Sept. 23, 2015 (Javers 2015). Francis also antagonized top clerics and Catholic moralists when he declared in a 2020 documentary entitled "Francesco," that gays are also God's children and are entitled to legal rights to civil marriage and family life in society (Horowitz 2020). Thus, one conservative bishop of Rhode Island, for instance, declared: "The pope's statement clearly contradicts what has been the long-standing teaching of the church about same-sex unions...The church cannot support the acceptance of objectively immoral relationships" (Winfield 2020, para.7).

Amid the growing social discrimination of nonbinary people in the Church and society, Pope Francis assured members of the LGBTQI community for greater ecclesial acceptance in the future. In his reply to a personal letter sent by a gay Catholic reporter who covers the church, he assured him of a dialogue between the LGBTQIcommunity and top members of the Catholic hierarchy in the future for greater LGBTQI integration in the RCC (O' Loughlin 2021).

However, progressive Catholics and scholars as well as LGBTQI leaders have sense some ambiguity in Pope Francis's welcoming attitude to the gay community in the Church and his conservative doctrinal stance on homosexuality. Despite his strong personal and pastoral care for homosexuals and members of the third sex in his public statements and writings, Francis remains faithful to the hostile doctrinal stance of the RCC towards homosexuality and transgenderism based on natural law theory, which as serious implication for the full inclusion of the LGBTQI community in the Church.

Francis still maintains the traditional church teaching founded on natural law that views homosexual attraction and deep-seated homosexual tendencies as naturally disordered and sinful (Catechism of the Catholic Church 1993, #2358). His welcoming attitude to members of the LGBTQI is unfortunately accompanied by a conservative doctrinal position based on natural law moral framework that philosophically judges homosexuality, "deep-seated" homosexual tendencies, and homosexual relationships as naturally disordered (Catechism of the Catholic Church 1993), a moral assessment that does not still incorporate the new findings of the social sciences regarding the nature of homosexuality (Shinnick 1997).

Pope Francis's showed mixed signals in his moral stance on homosexuality and ecclesial acceptance of nonbinary people in the RCC have bewildered both critics and progressive supporters. His strong compassion for gays and welcoming attitude for the LGBTQI in the Church is accompanied by a strong doctrinal stance that upholds the traditional natural law moral framework that frames the Catholic Church's moral teachings on homosexual orientation and behavior as unnatural and immoral. Thus, one wonders what keeps him to fully accept homosexuals and transgenders in the Christian community. Why did Francis label "gender' as an "ideology" rather than seeing it as an authentic human experience largely conditioned by society? Is gender a modern invention of feminism and LGBTQI movements of contemporary times?

This book primarily aims to address these questions. Some of its parts are based on the manuscripts of the book chapters I published in Springer Nature Singapore on gender ideology and LGBTQI inclusion in the Catholic Church. This volume aims to simplify the highly academic treatment of these chapters with the hope that the public can understand and appreciate their message in a less technical way. Academic publishing has its own jargons and norms, which are inappropriate for lay people. Thus, I revised, simplified, and self-published them to lower their price and thus accessible to the public as non-fiction books.

This volume contains three chapters. The first chapter provides a short introduction and short social background of the book. The second chapter sociologically clarifies whether the term "gender" as understood by the Catholic Church is an invention of LGBTQI and gay rights movements and feminism or it is truly an authentic human experience that dates to the origin of human civilization or since Adam and Eve or Adam and Steve. It also discusses homophobia and homophobic bullying and their consequences to the life the LGBTQI in the Church and society. Finally, it explores the promise of Pope Francis's concept synodality and inductive synodal theology to the full integration of the gay community in the Catholic Church.

The third chapter sociologically clarifies whether the concept of "gender" is a modern invention of feminist and LGBTQI movements in contemporary society as alleged by the Catholic Church and contemporary popes such as Pope Benedict XVI and Pope Francis. It also explains the difference between an ideology and sociological theory on gender. It argues that gender is an authentic human experience that dates back since the beginning of civilization and not a modern invention. Gender ideology is a misleading concept and a moral panic and exaggeration that discriminates the LGBTQI community in the Catholic Church. It proposes some alternative moral framework to welcome nonbinary Catholics in the Church.

The fourth chapter attempts to analyze the morality of sex change among transgender people in the Catholic Church, applying the inductive theological approach of Pope Francis and some tenets of the sociology of morality. It attempts to first analyze inductively the moral situation and societal context of sex change in today's contemporary world using the current sociological and social science research and literature before applying the Church's moral principles and making resolution on how the Catholic Church should deal guide Catholics on sex change and transgender sexuality.

Through this book, it is hoped that the Catholic Church and moral theologians would start to incorporate sociological and social science research on sexuality, gender, and gender diversity to update the ag-long natural law theory moral framework to fully welcome the LGBTQI community in the Church. The aim of this book is not to undermine the current Church moral doctrines but to find ways to adopt the sociological perspectives and research on gender and gender diversity in the Church's moral doctrines in response to the ecclesial call for all Catholics to inculturate the Church mission in contemporary society and to fully welcome the LGBTQI Catholics in the Christian community.

References

ABC News. 2014. "Leelah Alcorn: Transgender Teen's Reported Suicide Note Makes Dramatic Appeal." *ABC News Website* (31 December 2014). https://abcnews.go.com/US/leelah-alcorn-transgender-teens-reported-suicide-note-makes/story?id=27912326.

Catechism of the Catholic Church. 1993. Vatican: Libreria Editrice Vaticana. https://www.vatican.va/archive/ENG0015/_INDEX.HTM#fonte.

Fairchild, Phaylen. 2018. "Rejected in Death: When Families of Trans Suicide Victims Refuse to Acknowledge Their Gender." *Medium* (16 March 2018). https://phaylen.medium.com/rejected-in-death-when-families-of-trans-suicide-victims-refuse-to-acknowledge-their-gender-59b5e66a4efa.

Ford, Craig Jr. 2018. "Transgender Bodies, Catholic Schools, and a Queer Natural Law Theology of Exploration." *The Journal of Moral Theology* 7(1): 70-98.

Horowitz, J. 2020. "Pope Francis, in Shift for Church, Voices Support for Same Sex Civil Unions." *The New York Times.* (March 16, 2021). Available at https://www.nytimes.com/2020/10/21/world/europe/pope-francissame-sex-civil-unions.html

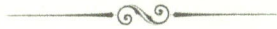

Javers, Eamon. 2015. "Pope Francis Met with Gay Couple Yayo Grassi and Iwan Bagus During His Time in U.S." NBC News (3 October 2025). https://www.nbcnews.com/storyline/pope-francis-visits-america/pope-francis-met-gay-couple-yayo-grassi-iwan-bagus-during-n437651

Navetta, Jean-Marie. [6]2014. "PFLAG executive: Most LGBTQ people see the Catholic Church as "unfriendly." What is our response?" Outreach (20 September 2022). https://outreach.faith/2022/09/pflag-executive-most-lgbtq-people-see-the-catholic-church-as-unfriendly-what-is-our-response/.

O'Loughlin, Michael. 2021. "Pope Francis Sent Me a Letter. It Gives Me Hope as a Gay Catholic." *International New York Times*, 17 Nov. 2021, p. NA. *Gale Academic OneFile*, link.gale.com/apps/doc/A682734143/AONE?u=anon~3064959a&sid=googleScholar&xid=d5d2bbc4. Accessed 15 June 2024.

---

6.   https://outreach.faith/
news-views/?_authors=cap-jean-marie-navetta&authors-nn=Jean-Marie%20Navetta

Winfield, Nicole.2020. "Francis Becomes 1st Pope to Endorse Same-Sex Civil Unions." *Associated Press* (21 October 2020). https://apnews.com/article/pope-endorse-same-sex-civil-unions-eb3509b30ebac35e91aa7cbda2013de2.

————— ⟨∾⟩ —————

Shinnick, Maurice. 1997. *The Remarkable Gift: Being Gay and Catholic*, Allen and Unwin, St. Leonards, NSW.

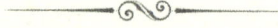

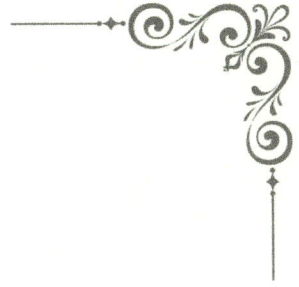

Chapter 2

Dignity, Transgenderism, Homophobia, and the LGBTQI
in the Catholic Church

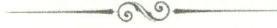

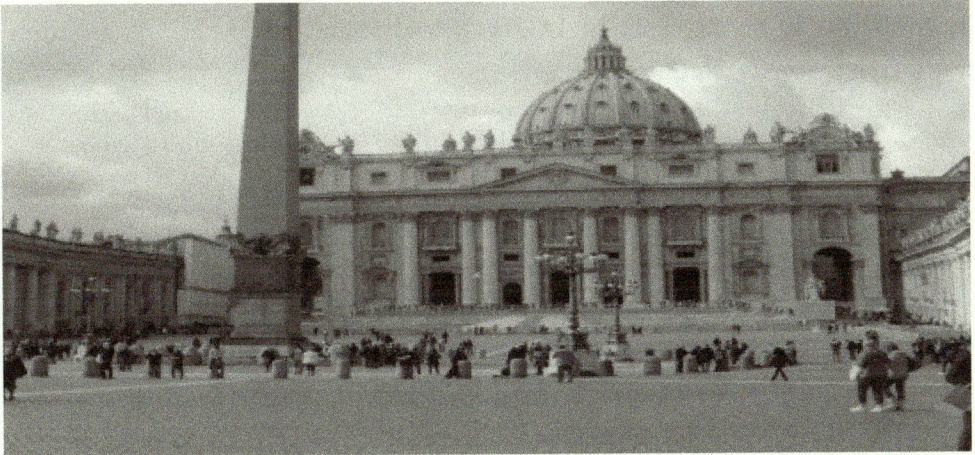

Photo: Vatican_rome_saint_peter.jpg **Credit:** Pixabay/Free-Images.com

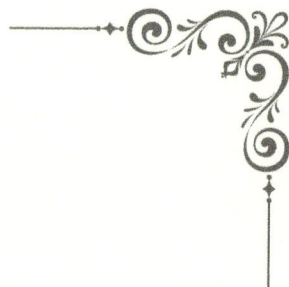

Introduction

When the Vatican released the Catholic Church's moral declaration *Dignitas Infinita* [Infinite Dignity] that condemned the criminalization of homosexuality, the LGBTQI community celebrates! (DDF 2024). But when it calls gender as an "ideology" and 'invention' as well as teaching that human dignity for persons as created in the image and likeness of God is only reserved to heterosexuals and biological males and females, the LGBTQI laments!

Reacted strongly against *Dignitas Infinita*'s characterization of human dignity that excludes transgenders and the LGBTQI, one retired Catholic deacon, who is an advocate of LGBTQI rights and the father of an adult transgender woman, claimed:

> While *Dignitas Infinita* begins by beautifully proclaiming our belief in the infinite dignity that every human person possesses, it then goes on to effectively deny that very dignity to transgender and gender diverse individuals. The document, and the five-year process that produced it, reflect a continuing stubborn refusal to engage with transgender people, the scientists and scholars who understand them best, and the medical community that provides them with the gender-affirming care they need to live. Denying transgender people access to gender-affirming care is tantamount to denying them any possibility of living with the human dignity that this document claims to uphold.[4]

Transgenders and nonbinary LGBTQI Catholics were bewildered by the document's exclusionary tone. They asked: How come that the Catholic Church, which they consider as their spiritual home, has rejected them as persons with infinite dignity? Why were they rejected by the document as people with human dignity? Is it because they happen to have non-heterosexual gender identities as gays, trans, queer, or members of the LGBTQI, which are not completely of their own choice but largely influenced by society and culture? Why are their gender considered an ideology and modern invention? As one transgender leader argues:

> Transgender people have existed throughout human history[1]—and we have been given places of honor in cultures that recognize our unique gifts. Yet we are often treated as a modern invention or as members of a group pushing an "ideology." This view of the transgender community both ignores history and glosses over the beautiful and unique diversity that we bring to the world just by being who we are, through our *imago Dei*, created "in the image of God." (Maxwell 2024, para. 5)

Transgenderism and gender diversity are not recent invention nor product of gay rights, feminism, and LGBQI movements as wrongly assumed by Catholic bishops and moral theologians. They have existed since Adam and Eve or Adam and Steve. Various cultures around the globe have acknowledged the existence of non-heterosexual genders and third sex and are even honors in their societies. Fluid and nonbinary gender identities and presentations can be found across all recorded history (Feinberg, 1996), but only in the past decade has the notion of gender fluidity attained wide familiarity.

Homosexuality and Transgenderism is as Old as Civilization

The rise of nonbinary genders and transgenders is not a new phenomenon. They are not recent creation of the LGBTQI community. Homosexuality and non-heterosexual genders are authentic human experience in various societies around the globe. The genders associated LGBTQI may be relatively modern to contemporary ears and homophobes, but ancient art and literature show that homosexual nonconforming behavior have occurred throughout history. A closer empirical scrutiny reveals that homosexuals, transgenders, or nonbinary people have long been existing since the time immemorial, albeit largely excluded and unrecognized in society.

---

1. https://www.nationalgeographic.com/history/article/how-historians-are-documenting-lives-of-transgender-people

"Throughout recorded history, homosexuals have comprised a small but significant cohort of society. Evidence of same-sex behavior dates to the oldest written texts, first noted in Egypt in 4,400 years ago, and subsequently found in ancient Greece, Rome, and China" (O' Keefe, O'Keefe, and Hodes 2018, 14). In India, for instance, the Hijas group has been recognized as the most typical third gender in Hindu culture for more than 2,000 years. People of nonbinary gender expression have been an important part of Hindu society since the ancien times. They are even mentioned in holy texts such as Ramayana and the Mahabharata with the hero Arjuna as the third gender to show their cultural significance.

Another example of a non-Western culture recognizing genders beyond heterosexuality is the Bugis tribe in South Sulawesi, Indonesia. It recognizes three gender categories beyond the binary. The first gender is the Calalai, which consists of individuals with female sexual characteristics but express themselves publicly in traditional masculine ways. The second is the Calabai gender, which includes individuals with male sexual characteristics and traditionally feminine expression. Lastly, the Bissu, which is a meta-gender group that manifests both masculine and feminine ways without identifying any of these traits.

. Cultural expressions of nonbinary sexuality have been recognized in non-Western cultures before the Catholic Church popularized "gender ideology", suggesting that nonbinary gender is not an invention. Before the rise of LGBTQI activism and pro-gender movements became popular in the contemporary world, gay and transgenders already existed. Sociologists, feminists, and other social scientists generally believe that various forms of non-heterosexual gender and homosexuality are not biological but social and cultural in nature (Sheldon et al. 2007). Only sex assigned during birth is biological.

Homosexuality and Transgender Identity as Social

The Catholic Church believes that homosexuality and transgenderism are purely a personal choice and a reflection of the current age that values absolute human freedom and expression. Pope Benedict XVI, for instance, considers homosexuality as a deviation of human sexuality and gender as ideology, a novel concept invented by feminists and gay activists. The lack sociological and social science academic training of Catholic clerics and sociologists as papal consultants are primarily a factor why gender and homosexuality tend to be seen as purely metaphysical and immutable. Educated in Scholastic philosophy and natural law moral framework, Catholic bishops and moral theologians cannot agree with social science research finding that gender is fluid, diverse, social, and cultural. One transgender aptly describes the gender of nonbinary people and gender diversity in society:

> Non-binary people are people who don't identify as male or female all the time. There are lots of subsections – you might be agender, gender fluid, bi-gender, a demi-girl or a demi-boy. You might not understand the nuances of the differences, but everyone is always making up new identities to match their experiences and that can only be a good thing. While it can be confusing, it's better than saying you can only be this thing, and we won't talk about anything else. (Lyons 2016, paras. 33)

Homosexuality and having a nonbinary gender are not totally the product of personal choice as wrongly assumed by the current teaching of the Church's catechism—that homosexuality is a sign of affective immaturity, applying the philosophical theory of natural law rather than the scientific method. Being a homosexual or member of the LGBTQI is not totally decided b he person. It is not only a matter of choosing what gender one wants to pursue as assumed by Church's teaching on gender but largely a social influence. As one lesbian confessed:

> From the age of about 5 yrs old till 15 yrs old I suffered from what is now being called 'gender dysphoria'. During this 10-year span of my life I experienced tremendous depression, I was unable to socially fit in with the other boys and girls my age. I just knew I was different and wasn't able to express why and I secretly carried this frustration till around the age of 15 yrs old when I discovered that my attraction to the same sex was not going to be solved by wishing and hoping that my body would magically change to male so that my attractions to girls would become socially acceptable. I discovered that perhaps I was a Lesbian. So, at 15 yrs old I made up my mind and lived as a closeted lesbian until I was outed at age 21.

Society and social interaction play a crucial and dominant role in shaping people's gender identity. That is why in behavioral sciences, gender is not metaphysical but social and cultural. It is greatly shaped by society and by immediate social environment where individuals developed their self and gender identity. In sociology, there is no such thing as absolute freedom. When people are born in society, they are thrown into a sea of social norms that restrict their choice. They are conditioned by social structure, that is, society's enduring and patterned behaviors learned through socialization process. Thus, it is sociologically wrong to assume that gender identity is purely a personal choice.

Immediately after this the release of *Dignitas Infinita*, a group of Catholic ministers, theologians, and students wrote an open letter in the media. This was addressed to Pope Francis who approved this document and to the Dicastery for the Doctrine of the Faith, the Vatican doctrinal watchdog, which prepared it, lamenting its lack of empathy and understanding of the lived gender experiences of the LGBTQI community in society. In his letter, they also expressed their fear that *Dignitas Infinita's* wrong characterization of gender as ideology would further expose gender-nonconforming Catholics to harm and victimization in society:

We read with gratitude the document's insistence on inalienable human dignity for migrants, the poor, and others whose dignity is consistently violated. We are saddened, therefore, that the document fails to recognize the dignity of trans and gender-nonconforming people. In its condemnation of gender "ideology" and "sex change," the document marginalizes the infinite dignity in people of all genders and their authentic self-expression and inadvertently perpetuates the harm it aims to overcome. [5]

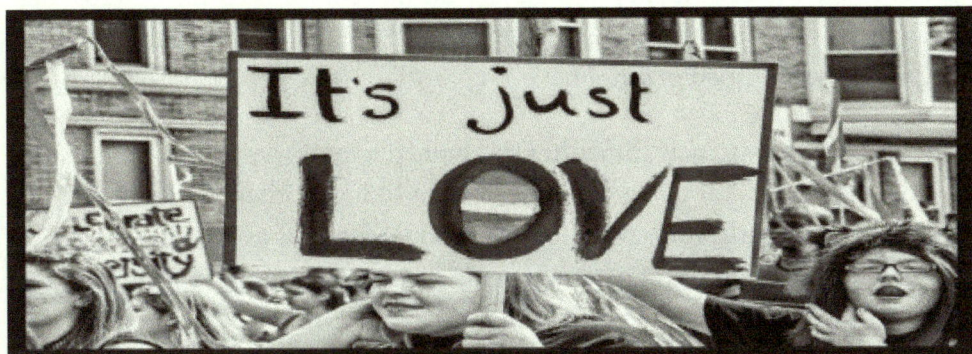

Photo: gay_pride_gay_gay.jpg **Credit:** Pixabay/Free-Images.com

The Co-Chair of Equal Voices[2], the national Australian ecumenical LGBTIQA+ organization, and Chair of Rainbow Catholics Inter agency Australia[3], Benjamin Oh (he/him), lamented *Dignitas Infinita's* lack of compassion for LGBTQI persons:

> The document clearly exposes the gap in the drafters' knowledge and understanding of LGBTQI realities. What is most saddening, however, is the document's lack of compassion for our trans, gender diverse and nonbinary siblings, demonstrated in how the authors write in dehumanizing, impersonal ways about that community, detached from their lived experiences. I am very concerned that this document will fuel more ignorance, violence, discrimination and abuse directed at LGBTQI people in our church and society, especially in communities where our trans, gender diverse, and nonbinary siblings are already attacked.[6]

The Real Concern: Homophobic and Transphobic Bullying

Being nonbinary and a member of the LGBTQI often results in homophobic and transphobic bullying. Homophobia or the fear of homosexuality and rigid heteronormativity that only recognizes heterosexuals as true human beings in society often lead to bullying. Gays and members of

2.   http://www.equalvoices.org.au/

3.   http://www.rainbowcatholics.com.au/

the LGBTQI whose sexuality and gender do not conform to the heterosexual standards are bullied in school, employment, and even in their churches.

One gay was bullied in school:

> School was extremely difficult. I got bullied a lot. I was picked on for being too thin, for being feminine, for not liking football, for hanging round with girls, for having long hair. They mocked everything they could think of in terms of gender and sexuality. (Lyons 2016, para.2)

A 19-year-old gay student in the Philippines, the world's third largest Catholic country, also narrated her experience of bullying:

> "When I was in high school, they'd push me, punch me. When I'd get out of school, they'd follow me [and] push me, call me 'gay,' 'faggot,' things like that." While verbal bullying appeared to be the most prevalent problem that LGBT students faced, physical bullying and sexualized harassment were also worryingly common—and while students were most often the culprits, teachers ignored or participated in bullying as well. The effects of this bullying were devastating to the youth who were targeted.[7]

Another transgender, a retired sales manager shared her painful experience of bullying and harassment:

> I had one job where they got rid of me and then they wrote to every company I applied to and said: "Don't employ this person, they're trans." Each time I lost my job we had to move. The last time it happened my wife wouldn't move any more – that's what really ended our marriage...When I transitioned full-time [in 2007] we had difficulties like having the car regularly damaged and having "the trannies live here" painted on the house. (Lyons 2016, paras. 29-30)

Homophobic Bullying in Religion

Transgenders are also ostracized in their own religions and churches. For example, a court ruling has denied a transgender woman to have a regular direct contact with her five children on the basis they might be shunned by their ultra-Orthodox Jewish community.

> The woman will be allowed only to send letters to her children, after a judge concluded there was a real chance of "the children and their mother being marginalized or excluded by the ultra-Orthodox community" if face-to-face contact were permitted.

> As a result of the ruling, her contact with each child will be limited to letters four times a year, with the suggestion that these could be sent to mark three Jewish religious holidays – Pesach, Sukkot and Hanukkah – and the children's birthdays. (Watt 2017, paras. 1-5).

In the Catholic Church, institutional homophobia and homophobic bullying are prevalent. Church authorities often contributed to this bullying. Pastoral letters and instructions of bishops in their dioceses and Catholic schools, for instance, often reject homosexual lifestyle and transgenderism. As an example, the Catholic Bishops of England and Wales issued a pastoral letter on gender, highlighting the Church's teaching that gender is biological and not a social construction. This document, which is entitled *Intricately woven by the Lord: A pastoral reflection on gender by the bishops of England and Wales*, emphasizes that all people are welcome in the Church, but also maintains that the sexual identity should be based on complementarity between male and female and one's biological sex. It rejected the idea of gender diversity and non-heterosexual identities of the LGBTQI. It teaches the value of the body and importance of sexual differentiation as male and female.[8]

Living a normal and moral homosexual life in the Catholic Church seems an impossible task under the ideal natural law moral framework that only sees gender as cisgender, that is, the person's expression of masculinity and femininity should only correspond to their biological sex assigned since birth as male and female. The adoption of the deductive natural law morality poses a serious obstacle to the moral recognition of homosexuality as a distinct gender identity and full acceptance of the LGBTQI in the Catholic Church. Traditional Church teaching on gender views homosexuality as a "sin against nature" (Sean 2015, 629).

Members of the third sex and the LGBTQI community are then obliged by the Catholic Church to live a "sexless" life, that is, a life of perpetual sexual abstinence, ignoring their human sexual needs. Homosexuals cannot further entertain their homosexual desires since their "deep-seated" homosexual tendencies are judged as intrinsically sinful under the Catholic Church's universal catechism (1993). They were told in several church pastoral care programs to be celibate and abstain from sex despite the fact the celibacy is a rare gift as acknowledged by Christ himself.

The *Catechism of the Catholic Church* (2003) defines homosexual attraction as "an exclusive or predominant sexual attraction toward persons of the same sex, (#2357)." Thus, homosexuals and their nonbinary sexuality and gender are unfortunately considered "objectively disordered" (#2358) and a sign of affective immaturity by Church moral guardians.

Because of their continued ecclesial exclusion, homosexuals and LGBTQI Catholics begin to see themselves as outsiders, alienated from their religious identity, and developing a negative view of their own gender identity. Social exclusion and fear did not only push them away from the Church but also cause great strain within their personality (Meer 2019). Research by Kite and Bryant-Lees (2016), for instance, high school and college homosexuals had trouble revealing their true gender identity to others for fear of rejection. Members of the LGBTQI community often experienced intense psychological traumas that could lead to church departure and higher risk of committing suicide.

The Trevor Research project (2020)[9] on the social exclusion of the LGBTQI group, for instance, showed that seventy-two percent of the transgender respondents felt uncomfortable or bullied in the Catholic Church or Catholic event because of their nonbinary gender. Sixty-four percent said that because of social exclusion being members of the LGBTQI group, they left the Church. Forty-six percent wanted emotional and psychological counselling for their mental anguish but unable to do so in the past twelve months. Finally, it revealed that 40 percent of transgender respondents had seriously considering suicide as well as inflecting self-harm for the past twelve months because of social exclusion and bullying.

Ultimately, it is homophobic and transphobic bullying in the Church and society that push transgender youth to commit suicide. Research showed that bullying of transgender teenagers often led to higher risk of suicide and self-harm. Suicide is said to be the worst consequence of homophobic bullying of the LGBTQI group in society. An earlier study by the Centers for Disease Control and Prevention (2015) among students in grades nine through 12, for example, revealed that 29 percent of the LGBTQI youth[4] had attempted suicide, compared with 9 percent of all students.

Fr. James Martin, S.J., a staunch LGBTQI defender in the Catholic Church, warned that issues of prejudice against the LGBTQI group are not just matters that affect church attendance but also life and death. Thus, he recommends building a bridge that can welcome the LGBTQI in the Catholic Church (Martin 2018). To Alison (2008), LGBTQI Catholics are generally treated as "they" rather than "you" by the Church hierarchy, making them outsiders rather than in insiders in the Christian community. This connection between social discrimination of the LGBTQI persons and higher risk of suicide is not only happening in the Catholic Church but also in other Christian denominations that perpetuate discriminatory practices that left transgenders without a spiritual home (Bockting and Cesaretti 2001).

Philosophical Lens of the Catholic Church on Gender

Why the Catholic Church remains indifferent to the unique gender experience of the LGBTQI community in the Church has something to do with philosophical moral lens used by Catholic bishops and theologians to understand gender and sexuality. The committee commissioned by the Catholic Church's Dicastery for the Doctrine of the Faith (DDF) to draft *Dignitas infinita* [Infinite Dignity] before Pope Francis approved it consisted mostly of philosophers and theologians with inadequate social science education and scientific knowledge on gender and sexuality.

The philosophical natural law moral framework on homosexuality as adopted by the Catholic Church is hostile to homosexuality as a distinct gender identity. The distinct gender identity and lifestyle of the LGBTQI have made gays and transgenders deviant and "immature" members in the eyes of the Church that used natural law gender framework. The Church moral magisterium or teaching office still teaches the Catholic faithful that heterosexuality is the

---

4.   https://www.cdc.gov/mmwr/volumes/65/ss/ss6509a1.htm

only gender standard for all Catholics. The traditional Thomistic understanding of natural law that strongly rejects any form of homosexual gender remains central to the official teaching of the Church's moral magisterium (Long 2013).

Using this philosophical framework of natural law, it is not surprising that *Dignitas Infinita* only conferred the ontological human dignity of Catholics heterosexuals as biological males and females. It is not also surprising that it only upholds the complementarity of sexes and labels "gender" as an ideology, implying that the diverse gender identity and nonbinary sexuality of the LGBTQI as unreal and mere social construction. The normative disciplines of Catholic philosophy and theology are largely responsible for his highly conceptual view of sex and gender as one, immutable, and inseparable realities ordained by God.

The philosophical theory of natural law, which originated from the pagan Stoic philosophy and popularized by St. Thomas Aquinas in the Catholic Church, remains the primary moral framework in Catholic morality on sexuality and gender. As the Catholic reporter Rebecca Weiss recalled his philosophy classes on sex and gender:

> In my college philosophy classes, I was taught that there can only be two sexes, that gender identity was based exclusively in biological sex, and that the male/female distinction was not only about physical characteristics but also about immutable essences of "masculine" and "feminine," rooted in the unchanging mind of God, and informing all of nature. (Weiss 2023, para.7).

Canonizing philosophical natural law moral framework since the Medieval times, the Catholic Church has stagnated its conceptual framework on sex and gender and rejected the sociological and scientific approaches to sexuality, gender, and gender diversity. It has not updated its traditional natural law moral framework, still maintaining the deductive reasoning to analyze Christian sexual morality despite the advent of inductive sociological and social science research on sex and gender; thus, the Church continues to ignore the lived experiences of nonbinary Catholics and the evolving gender diversity in society.

Thus, one nonbinary member of the German Catholic Church's Synodal Path process and queer rights activist named Mara Klein (they/them) expressed frustration with the Catholic Church's outdated views on gender diversity as reflected in *Dignitas Infinita*:

> Sadly, this new statement on gender studies and matters of gender diversity is very much in line with what we heard from the Vatican before. Yet again, the many voices of trans people of faith, as well as contemporary sciences are ignored completely in favor of an outdated, heteronormative, and self-referential anthropology.[10]

Transgenders and members of the LGBTQI community are regular and mature people in the Church and society. It is only homophobia that make them deviant and sub-human. They existed since Adam and Steve but were largely hidden in the closet because of the fear of homophobic and transphobic bullying. In the Catholic Church, for instance, gay priests are not only hidden in the closet or confessional box but in a cage. The Catholic Church blames gay priests as the primary sexual abusers in the Church despite scientific findings that should immature heterosexual priests as the main culprit.

By themselves, transgenders and members of the LGBTQI are normal people. They only become "abnormal" when homophobes and heterosexuals would tell them that they are not "normal." As one transgender psychology student narrated about how she felt about herself:

> On a day-to-day basis I don't tell people I'm transgender. The thing about trans people is, we feel very normal. It's the way we are, it's only when people say you're not normal that you feel that way.

> I've always been extremely feminine, I always felt that way. I can't say that I ever felt like a boy, I just had to live as a boy for the first 16 years of my life. Trans people are the same as everyone else, our ideals in life are to be happy, to be respected, to be comfortable. I've had people who have openly said to me that they've had prejudices around trans people but as soon as they've met me, they've understood more – it's who I am and the way that I was born. There's no real difference between myself and people who are cisgender [non-transgender]. (Lyons 2016, paras. 5-7)

According to one transgender, Surat-Shaan Knan, 40s, project manager for Liberal Judaism, London, no one should dictate another person how he or she tell how one should live his or life and identity:

> I don't think anyone should be able to tell you who you are and how to live your life. Yourself is yourself, even in the religious community.

Being a non-heterosexual with nonbinary sexuality and gender is not invented; it is socially learned in one's culture and social environment. It is wrong and inaccurate to say that the members of LGBTQI group just woke and decided to be non-heterosexual. No. It is largely unintentional and product of social interaction during their formative years as children and adolescents that nonbinary gender and sexuality are constituted in one's personality and identity. A person cannot become a gay or transgender since birth alone. Gender is relational. It is always formed in relation to others especially during the formative years. As one transgender recalled:

> Until I was about four or five, I didn't know I wasn't a girl, to be honest with you. One of my earliest memories, about five years old, was being yelled at by a teacher for going to the toilet with the girls. About the same age I realized I was different to these other boys. At the age of nine I refused to have my hair cut. I didn't have it cut until I was 16, because having it cut was such a torment to me. (Lyons 2016, para.1)

Pope Francis and the LGBTQI

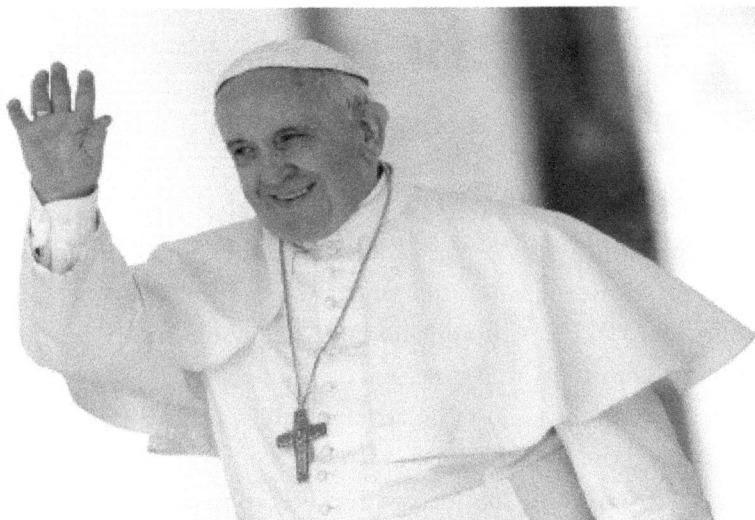

Photo: Pope Francis **Credit:** Flickr/Free-Images.com

———— ❧ ————

The election of Cardinal Jorge Bergoglio as Pope Francis in 2013 promises a new attitude of the Catholic Church towards the LGBTQI community. One of the hallmarks of Francis's pontificate is his strong compassion and pastoral concern for the marginalized and socially discriminated people in society such as the nonbinary members of the LGBTQI community.

No other popes in Church history who has shown great love for homosexual and transgender Catholics and their social and spiritual integration in the Catholic Church than Francis. His liberal and friendly stance towards gays, as shown in his media pronouncements and writings, has put him at odds with conservative clerics, Catholics, and critics in the Catholic Church to the extent of accusing him of schism, blasphemy, and heresy.[11]

Despite this, Pope Francis's have shown mixed signals on his moral stance on homosexuality and ecclesial acceptance of nonbinary people in the Catholic Church, which bewildered both critics and progressive supporters. His strong compassion for gays and welcoming attitude towards the LGBTQI in the Church is accompanied by a strong doctrinal stance that upholds the traditional natural law moral framework that frames the Catholic Church's moral teachings on homosexual orientation and gender diversity as unnatural and immoral.

In his media pronouncements and writings, Francis still maintains the Church's philosophical moral framework that only allows heterosexuality as the only gender norm in the Church to frame his LGBTQI inclusion in the Catholic Church. Like his predecessors Pope John Paul II and Pope Benedict XVI, he remains steadfast in his strong belief that changing one's sex and gender assigned during birth is contravening the natural complementarity of sexes ordained by God (Francis 2015). Although he endorsed same-sex civil union, he remains opposed to the sacramental marriage of gay couples despite his approval of their pastoral blessing by priests in the Church declaration *Fiducia Supplicans* [Supplicating Trust] (DDF 2023).

To Francis, all talks about gender alteration and diversity in society that oppose heterosexuality and gender complementarity of sexes are collectively labelled as "gender ideology," which he sees as an ideological colonization of the West (Patternote and Kuhar 2017; Case 2019), an imposition of decadent Western values of developed countries on developing nations. He resists seeing homosexuality as a distinct sexual orientation and gender identity like heterosexuals in the Catholic Church.

Thus, Francis still maintains the traditional moral teaching that "deep-seated homosexual tendencies" and sexual acts are sinful and naturally disordered according to the natural law morality of the Church (Catechism of the Catholic Church 1993, #377-378). As Millies (2023, para.7) argues:

> The pope's support for LGBTQ people's civil rights does not change Catholic doctrine about marriage or sexuality. The church still teaches – and will certainly go on teaching – that any sexual relationship outside a marriage is wrong, and that marriage is between a man and a woman. It would be a mistake to conclude that Francis is suggesting any change in doctrine.

Following his predecessor Pope Benedict XVI, Pope Francis labels the contemporary concept of gender and gender theory as "gender ideology." Benedict XVI is said to play a key role in the adoption, circulation, and legitimation of this term in the RCC (Vaggione 2020). His reading of the antifeminist pamphlet of the American journalist-activist Dale O' Leary entitled "Gender: The Deconstruction of Women" has allegedly influenced his negative attitude towards feminism and gender theories (Graff 2016).

The term "gender ideology" originated within Catholicism (Vaggione 2020). "Gender theory" and "gender ideology" are terms "invented" within the Catholic Church through Pope Benedict XVI to understand and counter the influence of the feminist and LGBTQI movements, which were growing in popularity in the United States, Europe, and Latin America. Gender ideology" became a concept, a signifier for perceived evils of liberalism in the realm of human sexuality by conservative Catholics.

Pope Francis adopted the concept of gender as an ideology from Pope Benedict XVI and gave it a new visibility to anti-gender movements by calling it as an "ideological colonization" (Francis 2015). To Francis, gender ideology is a "neocolonial project through which Western activists and their governments try to export their decadent values and secularize non-Western societies" (Patternote and Kuhar 2017, 8) concerning gender, gender diversity, transgender sexuality, non-traditional forms of family structure, and other perceived anti-Catholic moral concerns. Indeed, Pope Francis has provided new "tactics and strategies for this war, with his rhetoric of anticolonialism and his combination of warm receptivity to individuals with continuing opposition to their rights" (Case 2019, 659).

An ideology is a set of ideas that interpret history. It is an ideal reality that aims to conform all human experiences according to its vision of social reality. An ideology therefore is not the empirical world that people live today but an ideal world in which the ideologues or people who promote it aimed to achieve in society. As Millies (2014, para. 8) argues:

> What is essential about an ideology is that it must be false. That is to say, an ideology rejects the reality that does not correspond to an idea. An ideology begins with an idea that is contrary to reality, and then makes reality fit with that idea—which always demands force. (Millies 2014, para. 8)

So, if gender is perceived by Pope Francis and the Catholic Church as an ideology rather than a social reality, then it is not understood as culturally and historically real but false. Thus, the genders and gender diversity of the LGBTQI that deviate from heterosexuality and gender complementarity of male and female as the only gender norms in society as taught by the Church is false. For Francis, the gender diversity of the LGBTQI remains merely a social construction, invention, and imposition by Western countries largely influenced by feminism, political right, as well as gay rights movement and activism.

Seeing gender as a social construction and an ideology in the Catholic Church moral teaching is the primary objection of sociologists, feminists, and LGBTQI leaders who view it as social and cultural experience. Gender for the LGBTQI is an authentic human experience, fluid, and diverse, which cannot be reduced to heterosexuality and gender complementarity.

Despite Francis's rejection of gender as an authentic human experience but as an invention and ideology, a dawn and silver lining for the LGBTQI inclusion in the Catholic Church can be expected from him with his new ecclesial process called synodality and inductive synodal theology that first requires inductive knowing of people's lived experiences before moral and theological reflection and judgment.

The Promise of Pope Francis for Greater Inclusivity

In his apostolic exhortation *Evangelii Gaudium* [The Joy of the Gospel] (EG), Pope Francis (2013) admitted that the church hierarchy needs to be in dialogue with other voices, including those who disagree with church teaching. He recognized that the Catholic Church has no monopoly of all truths. Thus, he encourage a fruitful dialogue between Catholic theology and other academic disciplines as necessary to understand difficult moral issues such as gender, homosexuality, and LGBTQI inclusivity in the Church. Following the spirit of EG, McCarty (2015, 10) aptly argues:

> Dialogue with the Catholic Church on the matter of gender and sexual diversities must draw attention to this change in church teaching as a doorway to more fruitful dialogue with the church on the social and moral status of same-sex activities. While church teachers may front the official moral dogma on homosexual orientation as "a disposition ordered toward intrinsic moral evil," and same-sex activity as "gravely disordered and contrary to nature," we

must ask—in the spirit of *Evangelii Gaudium*—that this dogma be put in a dialogical relationship with the social and natural sciences, as well as with works in the humanities (especially ethics), that demonstrate how homosexual orientation and same-sex activities can—by the light of prudence—contribute to human flourishing....(McCarty 2015, 10).

Indeed, Pope Francis does not intend to eschew church teaching. One cannot expect him "to suddenly change course from its long-held procreative and marital norms in relation to its moral theology of sex and sexuality. However, Francis's leadership suggests a change of both tone and mediation of conflict" (McCarty 2015, 4). "What is striking about Pope Francis is not that he is revising dogma or undoing the hierarchy...Rather, Francis appears to be applying a more prudential and pastoral approach to church orthodoxy than what his predecessor did" (McCarty 2014, para. 4).

Pope Francis's inductive synodal theology in his short document known as *Ad Theologiam Promovendam* [To Promote Theology] is calling for a paradigm shift in Catholic theology that requires an scinetific inductive approach, needing an accurate understanding of people's lived experiences as the starting point before theological reflection (Francis 2023). Thus, it implies the utilization of scientific research about people's concrete experiences before theologizing or applying theoretical interpretation such as the gender experiences of the LGBTQI Catholics.

Pope Francis's inductive synodal approach coincides with the inductive scientific research of sociology and other social sciences that typically begins with data collection and ends up applying a particular appropriate theory to interpret them. In the grounded theory approach, for instance, the theory may emanate from the patterns of the data collected by the investigator to understand the empirical reality. An inductive synodal-sociological moral framework is more appropriate framework than the current philosophical natural law to fully accept the LGBTQI Catholics in the Church today.

The Catholic Church should then listen from people from below, especially to those in the peripheries such as sociologists, feminists, and gender advocates whose approach is often labelled as "scientism" and thus unheard and condemned in the Church. Francis's Synod on inductive synodal process implies consultation and listening to the LGBTQI community and learning from people behind "gender ideology" to achieve a more inclusive synodal church, a church that welcomes the voiceless and marginalized in society such as the LGBTQI group.

References

Alison, J. 2008. Letter to a Young Gay Catholic." *James Alison Theology Website* (20 January 2008. https://jamesalison.com/letter-to-a-young-gay-catholic/.

Bockting, Walter O., and Charles Cesaretti. 2001. "Spirituality, Transgender Identity, and Coming Out." *Journal of Sex Education and Therapy* 26 (4): 291–300. https://doi.org/10.1080/01614576.2001.11074435.

Case, Mary Anne. 2019. "Trans Formations in the Vatican's War on "Gender Ideology." *Signs: Journal of Women in Culture and Society* 44(3): 639-664.

Catechism of the Catholic Church. 1993. Vatican: Libreria Editrice Vaticana. https://www.vatican.va/archive/ENG0015/_INDEX.HTM#fonte.

Corrêa, Sonia. 2017. Gender Ideology: tracking its origins and meanings in current gender politics[5]. LSE Blogs (11 December 2017).

DDF (Dicastery of the Doctrine of the Faith). 2023. "On the Pastoral Meaning of Blessings." Vatican: The Roman Curia. Available at: https://www.vatican.va/roman_curia/congregations/cfaith/documents/rc_ddf_doc_20231218_fiducia-supplicans_en.html

DDF (Dicastery of the Doctrine of the Faith). 2024. "Declaration *Dignitas Infinita* on Human Dignity. Vatican: The Roman Curia. https://www.vatican.va/roman_curia/congregations/cfaith/documents/rc_ddf_doc_20240402_dignitas-infinita_en.html.

Feinberg, Leslie. 1996. *Transgender Warriors: Making History from Joan of Arc to Dennis Rodman*. Boston, MA: Beacon Press.

Francis. 2013. *Evangelii Gaudium* [The Joy of the Gospel]: *An Apostolic Exhortation on the Proclamation of the Gospel in Today's World*. Vatican: Dicastero per la Comunicazione - Libreria Editrice Vaticana https://www.vatican.va/content/francesco/en/apost_exhortations/documents/papa-francesco_esortazione-ap_20131124_evangelii-gaudium.html

---

5.   https://blogs.lse.ac.uk/gender/2017/12/11/gender-ideology-tracking-its-origins-and-meanings-in-current-gender-politics/

Francis. 2015. "*Laudato Si*: Pope Francis's Encyclical on the Care of Our Common Home." Vatican: Dicastero per la Comunicazione - Libreria Editrice Vaticana.

Francis. 2023. "Apostolic Letter Issued "Motu Proprio" *Ad Theologiam Promovendam.*" Vatican. Unofficial English translation available at: https://www.vatican.va/content/francesco/en/events/event.dir.html/content/vaticanevents/en/2023/11/1/ad-theologiam-promovendam.html.

Gallo, Michelle. 2017. "Gender Ideology" Is a Fiction That Could Do Real Harm." *Open Society Foundations* (29 August 2017). https://www.opensocietyfoundations.org/voices/gender-ideology-fiction-could-do-real-harm.

Graff, Agnieszka. 2016. "'Gender Ideology': Weak Concepts, Powerful Politics." *Religion and Gender* 6(2): 268-272. https://doi.org/10.18352/rg.10177

Kuzma, Maxwell. 2024." As a transgender Catholic, I don't see gender diversity as a threat to our faith." Outreach (10 April 2024). https://outreach.faith/2024/04/as-a-transgender-catholic-i-dont-see-gender-diversity-as-a-threat-to-our-faith/

Long, Steven A. 2013. "Fundamental Errors of the New Natural Law Theory." *The National Catholic Bioethics Center* 13(1): 105-131.

Lyons, Kate. 2016." Transgender stories: 'People think we wake up and decide to be trans.' The Guardian (10 July 2016). https://www.theguardian.com/society/2016/jul/10/transgender-stories-people-think-we-wake-up-and-decide-to-be-trans.

Mackay, Finn. 2024. "'Gender ideology' is all around us – but it's not what the Tories say it is." *The Guardian* (19 January 2014).

Martin, James S.J. 2018. *Building a Bridge: How the Catholic Church and the LGBT Community Can Enter Into a Relationship of Respect, Compassion, and Sensitivity.* Revised Expanded Edition. San Francisco, CA: Harper One.

McCarty, Richard. 2014. "Objects of the Inquisition." *Academe Blog* (17 January 2014). https://academeblog.org/2014/01/17/more-about-objects-of-the-inquisition/

Millies, Steven P. 2023. "It Shouldn't Seem So Surprising When the Pope Says Being Gay 'Isn't A Crime' – A Catholic Theologian Explains." *The Conversation* (26 January 2023).

O' Keefe, James, O' Keefe, Evan, and Hodes, John. 2018. "Evolutionary Origins of Homosexuality." *The Gay & Lesbian Review* (January-February 2018): 14-18.

Paternotte, David, and Kuhar, Roman. 2017. "Chapter 1: "'Gender Ideology' in Movement: An Introduction."" In Roman Kuhar and David Paternotte, eds, *Anti-gender campaigns in Europe: Mobilizing Against Equality,* 1– 22. New York, London: Rowman & Littlefield International.

Philips, S.U. 2001. "Gender Ideology: Cross-cultural Aspects." In Neil J. Smelser, Paul B. Baltes, (eds). *International Encyclopedia of the Social & Behavioral Sciences,* 6016-6020. Pergamon.

Reid, Graeme. 2018. 'Breaking the Buzzword: Fighting the "Gender Ideology" Myth.' *Human Rights Watch* (10 December 2018).

Sheldon JP, Pfeffer CA, Jayaratne TE, Feldbaum M, and Petty EM. 2007. "Beliefs About the Etiology of Homosexuality and About the Ramifications of Discovering its Possible Genetic Origin. *Journal of Homosexuality* 52(3-4):111-50. https://doi.org/10.1300/J082v52n03_06. PMID: 17594974; PMCID: PMC4545255.

Vaggione, Jun Marco. 2020. "The Conservative Uses of Law: The Catholic Mobilization Against Gender Ideology" *Social Compass* 2020 67(2) 252–266. https://doi.org/10.1177/0037768620907561   journals.sagepub.com/home/scp.

Watt, Holly. 2017. Transgender woman denied contact with her ultra-Orthodox Jewish children. The Guardian (30 January 2017). https://www.theguardian.com/society/2017/jan/30/transgender-woman-denied-direct-access-to-ultra-orthodox-jewish-children.

Weiss, Rebecca B. 2023." The Catholic Church's gender ideology is complementarian and binary. That's not how nature works. The National Catholic Reporter (24 April 2023). https://www.ncronline.org/opinion/ncr-voices/catholic-churchs-gender-ideology-complementarian-and-binary-thats-not-how-nature.

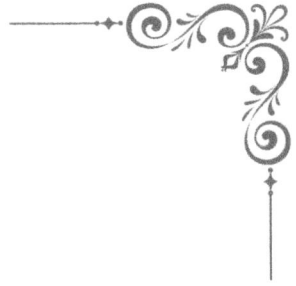

Chapter 3

Is Gender an Invention or Authentic Human Experience?

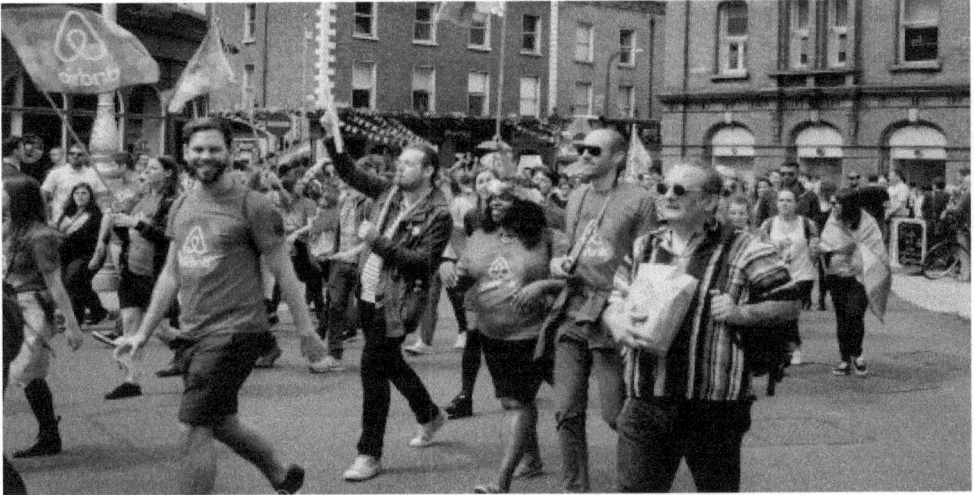

Photo: dublin_lgbtq_pride_parade_27.jpg **Credit:** Flickr/Free-Images.com

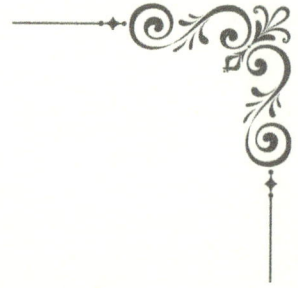

Introduction

Sociologists and social scientists believe that there are more than two genders in the world that are traditionally understood as straight people who are biologically male and female. Heterosexuality has always been the general gender norm in most societies around the globe. Although they constitute a minority in society, there are also non-heterosexuals or those who constitute the lesbian, gay, bisexual, transgender, queer, and intersexual (LGBTQI) community who also exist in several societies as regular persons. Being a minority in society, nonbinary people who experience discrepancy between their assigned sex since birth and their experience of masculinity and femininity, are often harassed and bullied for being different in gender identity.

Sociologists of gender generally agree that there are various forms of nonbinary sexualities in the world, and that homosexuality is not biological but social and cultural (Sheldon et al. 2007). Thus, the rise of transgenderism and nonbinary genders in society. Transgenderism and gender diversity are concepts that recognize the existence of several evolving forms of genders in the world as well as nonbinary or non-heterosexual people in the planet. It is not something that is invented or started by feminist and gay rights movements and LGBTQI activism in the Western world as assumed by recent papal teachings.

Cultural expressions of nonbinary sexuality are already recognized in non-Western cultures before the advent of LGBTQI activism, gay rights movements, and feminism in the contemporary world. Scientists generally believe that there is no specific gene that associates it to homosexuality and nonbinary genders to date. Researchers have not identified credible linkages to any genetic region in lesbians for instance (Veniegas and Conley 2000[1]). Findings from genetic studies of homosexuality in humans have been

---

1.   https://www.ncbi.nlm.nih.gov/pmc/articles/PMC4545255/#R81

confusing—contradictory at worst and tantalizing at best—with no clear, strong, compelling evidence for a distinctly genetic basis for homosexuality.

The Catholic Church believes that sex and gender are inseparable, ahistorical, and metaphysically ordained by God, contrary to the sociological and social science research. Interpreting the Book of Genesis literally that God created a man and a woman, the Church teaches that the only the gender norm in society is heterosexuality and gender complementarity of sexes, rejecting all beliefs about gender diversity. For Catholic bishops and moral theologians, those who advocate gender and gender diversity are influenced by what they labelled as "gender ideology" of the West that invents the existence of nonbinary or non-heterosexual genders such as those of the LGBTQI community.

Pope Benedict XVI popularized the concept of "gender ideology" within the Catholic Church. After reading the anti-feminist writing of the American journalist-activist Dale O' Leary entitled "Gender: The Deconstruction of Women," Benedict XVI formed a negative attitude towards feminism and gender theories (Graff 2016). He then played a key role in the adoption, circulation, and legitimation of this misleading concept "gender ideology" in the Catholic Church (Vaggione 2020), which sees gender as an invention and mere influence of feminism and LGBTQI movement rather than an authentic human experience.

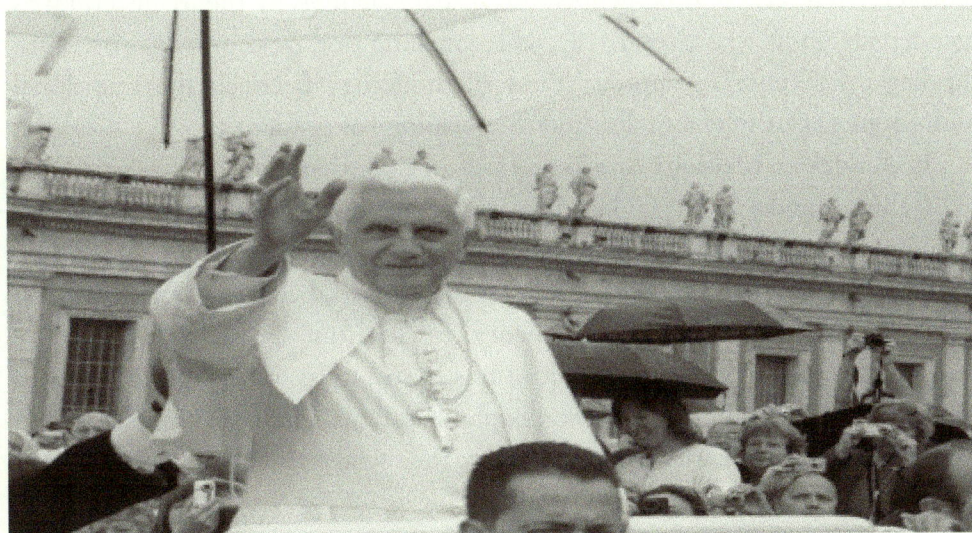

Photo: benedykt_xvi.jpg **Credit**: Wikimedia/Free-Images.com

Following Benedict XVI, Pope Francis also labels gender as an ideology. To him, the contemporary concept of gender espoused by feminists, sociologists, and LGBTQI leaders is a modern invention. It is an ideology that threatens the very survival of humanity, which consist only of biological males and females as planned and taught by God in human creation. That is why for Francis, gender is a form of colonization of advanced Western countries, an imposition of decadent moral values on developing countries. It is only part of a Western neocolonial project by gender activists and their governments (Patternote and Kuhar 2017).

In an interview[2] with the Argentine daily newspaper *La Nación* [The Nation] last March 10, 2023, Francis reiterated the exaggeration of gender as "gender ideology" which he considered as the "most dangerous" one today (Mares 2023). He also labelled gender as "ugliest ideology of our time" because it cancels all distinctions between a man and a woman (Zengarini 2024). To him, "God created man and woman; God created the world in a certain way... and we are doing the exact opposite...This is the age of sin against God the Creator" (Francis 2016, *para.* 42).

Because of the strong influence of the theology of the body espoused by Pope John Paul II and reaffirmed by Pope Benedict XVI, Pope Francis and the Catholic Church have inappropriately classified all sociological and social science perspectives on gender and gender diversity that tend to oppose the official church teachings on gender and sexual teachings by the Magisterium as "gender ideology" (Ford Jr. 2018). This labelling does acknowledge, however, the basic difference in approach and methodology between the traditional philosophical Catholic morality and the sociology of gender.

Is Gender an Ideology or a True Human Experience?

Calling gender and gender theories as the ugliest and most dangerous ideology of the times runs counter to the scientific gender approaches of modern sociology and the social sciences. Gender sociologists, behavioral scientists, and feminists basically view gender theory in scientific research as tentative explanations of the various gender relations in society as well as social injustices against women and gender-diverse people in today's world that are subject to data confirmation. Gender as understood in the social sciences is not an ideology

---

2.   https://www.lanacion.com.ar/el-mundo/entrevista-de-la-nacion-con-el-papa-francisco-la-ideologia-del-genero-es-de-las-colonizaciones-nid10032023/

but a true human experience in society. An ideology consists of ideal beliefs about society, which do not necessarily reflect reality.

To Philips (2001, 6016), the term 'ideology' reflects "two aspects of research on this topic: (a) its roots in the feminist position that women are conceptualized as inferior to men to justify and sustain social and cultural systems dominated by men; and (b) the culturally constructed (as opposed to 'natural') nature of gender." The concept of "gender ideology" is actually "nothing to do with gender, as in masculinity and femininity, and how this shapes our identities. Instead, it is used to imply that trans, transgender and gender non-conforming identities are a new fad, and that the longstanding social justice movement for trans rights is really a recent conspiracy of nefarious elites[3] (Mackay 2024, para. 3).

"Like its buzzword brother "fake news," "gender ideology" hasn't taken long crossing borders into nationalist lexicons. The vacuous but dangerous term was adopted by the Holy See[4] decades ago to refer to a supposed gay and feminist-led movement to subvert traditional families and social values, a reaction against the rights of women and expanding protections for sexual and gender minorities" (Reid 2018, paras 2-3). Corrêa (2017) argues that the term "gender ideology" has no academic or theoretical basis, nor a clear and coherent definition:

[T]he semantic frame 'gender ideology' reveals itself as an empty and adaptable signifier, encompassing a broad range of demands such as the right to abortion, sexual orientation and gender identity, to diverse families, education in gender and sexuality, HIV prevention and sex work, a basic basket that can be easily adjusted to the conditions of each context. Its discourses construct unusual analogies between feminism, queer theory and communism, a strategy that has echoes in contexts where this spectrum remains active....

Mackay (2024, para. 4) also argues that:

Gender[5] ideology is real, but it wasn't invented by trans men or trans women, and it doesn't just apply to trans or transgender people. The

---

3.   https://freedomnews.org.uk/2019/06/16/gender-ideology-up-yours/

4.   https://chicagounbound.uchicago.edu/journal_articles/9669/

real gender ideology is the binary sex and gender system that requires all of us to be either male-masculine-heterosexual or female-feminine-heterosexual; and which attaches harsh penalties to those who deviate from this script.

So, what the Catholic Church and recent popes are teaching is all about the ideal "gender ideology" that all people should conform to the Biblical teaching on the natural complementarity of sexes as male and female, painting an ideal world rather than acknowledging that gender diversity exists since the beginning of time. As mentioned, an ideology is a set of ideal beliefs of what society ought to be rather than an accurate description of social reality such as the Marxist ideology of a classless society. Thus, the "gender ideology" is the Church's teaching on heteronormativity and not the gender diversity advocated by sociologists of gender, feminists, and members of the LGBTQI.

The papal teaching on "gender ideology" is actually the opposite of the empirical reality that shows diversity of genders beyond heterosexuality. That is why social scientists and feminists believe in gender fluidity and continuing evolution of genders in the contemporary world. Thus, the evolving acronym LGBTQI$^+$ or LGBTQIA$^+$ and their plus sign to indicate that there will more forms of gender in the future depending on the evolution of society that influences human sexuality and gender identity.

Is Gender Theory the Same as Gender Ideology?

Owing to the lack of sociology and social science training of Catholic clerics, Pope Benedict XVI and Pope Francis seem to confuse "gender theory" as an ideology. They also view gender as a social construction of the LGBTQI community rather than an authentic human experience. This is understandable since Catholic popes are also educated in philosophy and theology, lacking sociological training. They are not also surrounded by sociologists and gender specialists to advise them on gender matters but philosophers and theologians who view gender as metaphysical and based on the philosophical theory of natural law.

Following Benedict XVI and church tradition, the Catholic Church still maintains the philosophical approach to morality based on natural law theory,

---

5. https://www.theguardian.com/world/gender

disregarding most scientific research on complex moral issues of gender, gender diversity, transgenderism, or LGBTQI inclusivity. Sociological and feminist gender theories that aim to account gender relations and women's oppression in society as well as the emergence of gender diversity in society are often seen as opposing church moral doctrines and labelled as "gender ideology."

Instead of understanding the true nature of these scientific and sociological theories as part of scientific rationality that applies both theory and method or data collection to explain the nature of gender and gender relations in the world, the Church sees them as deviating from the philosophical reasoning of natural law and constituting an ideology. In sociology, a theory is still tentative and subject to data confirmation, thus not definitive; thus, labelling gender theories as an ideology that attacks church teaching is highly inaccurate that needs sociological clarification.

With the increasing cultural revolution of modern and contemporary societies, gender and sexuality can become more complex for Catholic hierarchy and moral theologians to understand without the assistance of sociologists and behavioral scientists on the evolving moral situations of gender. Currently, the emergence of gender research has become a major field in sociology. Sociological research on gender has had major impact in academic fields, specifically "in the education and health sectors, in violence prevention, antidiscrimination and equal opportunity policy" (Connell 2014, 550).

One serious problem associated with the use of "gender ideology" as a signifier for the Catholic Church against feminism and gender theory is its lack of distinction between an ideology and a theory. In sociology, there is a big difference between these two terms. An ideology carries a reformist stance of changing society according to a set of ideal beliefs about social reality, whereas a sociological theory, which also consists of beliefs and a set of principles but intends to describe or explain a social phenomenon based on a set of quantitative and/or qualitative data.

The use of theory to interpret data in sociological research is an essential component of modern sociology. Catholic philosophy and theology as normative disciplines adopt a theory to explain social reality but are not required to gather scientific data to support their theoretical explanation in empirical reality. To understand gender and gender relations in society, Catholic moral theologians fundamentally apply a deductive philosophical approach that applies the natural law theory without the need of a set of empirical data to ground their moral analysis.

The relationship between ideology and sociology is not an easy one". In sociology, ideology is generally seen as a set of beliefs that aim to explain and change social reality. It can be understood as a relatively coherent body of beliefs about the various aspects of society, that is, as a cultural system and a guide for policy. It has an activist aspiration of changing certain aspects of society for a certain social value or policy.

Gender as the person's expression of masculinity, femininity, and identity is vastly different from an ideology. Gender is an authentic human experience while ideology is a utopian reality or aspiration of what society should be according to its set of principles. Sociologists view gender as true human experience by nonbinary people and members of the LGBTQI community in the constantly evolving society, not a metaphysical reality as the Catholic Church understands. They also view gender theories as tools for research and social change to achieve societal reforms and social justice—a cause that is within the purview of the Catholic Church's social doctrines and Francis's synodal priorities of protecting the human dignity of the downtrodden in society (Ballano 2024).

The Church's set of beliefs about heteronormativity and gender complementarity is actually an ideology since it points to an ideal world where people should all be heterosexuals to be God's children with infinite human dignity. Gender as understood in sociology and feminism points to the empirical reality—that it is a social and cultural experience which evolves in time. It is not empirically true that people's gender always corresponds to their biological sex assigned since birth or cisgender. Nonbinary or non-heterosexual gender exists where sex as a biological reality and gender as a social experience disconnects resulting in transgenderism and homosexuality.

Gender sociological research acknowledges that there are various forms of gender beyond heterosexual model since the beginning of time. Historically, the distinction between sex and gender was proposed by gender studies in the 1970s. Since then, the term "gender" as not primarily referring to biological sex as being male or female but social and cultural constructions of masculinities and femininities. Recent gender studies suggest that gender identity is changing and can be performed or experienced in various ways. As Fontanella, Maretti, and Sarra (2014, 2553) contend:

Gender identity relies on a person's sense of self as male or female or feeling between sexes. The concept of gender identity can be better understood keeping distinguished the notions of "sex", "sexuality" and "gender". Even if gender seems to flow naturally from biological sex, gender and sex are not interchangeable terms. While sex principally refers to the biological aspects of male or female, being related to their physical anatomy (sex chromosomes, gonads, sex hormones, internal reproductive structures and external genitalia), gender includes, in addition to the biological elements, the behavioral, psychological and social characteristics of men and women.

Gender identity is the person's intrinsic self-identification of personal femaleness and maleness and his or her genitalia or biological traits assigned during birth. Using a naturalist and empirical explanation, gender in the social sciences is understood a social and cultural construction in society (Scott 1999). According to Deutsch (2007), gender is an ongoing emergent aspect of social interaction. It is not something that we are but something that we do (West and Zimmerman 1987).

Thus, contrary to the Catholic Church's conception of gender as immutable, ahistorical, and divinely ordained, social scientists, following methodological naturalism, that is, suspending personal biases such as religious belief of God as the creator to achieve a scientific understanding of the empirical reality, view gender as continuously changing and socially constructed by people across "time, cultures, contexts, ethnic groups and social situations" (Fontanella, Maretti, and Sarra 2014, 2553). It is evolving depending on the sociological and historical contingencies.

Gender diversity is continuously existing in the world and experienced by nonbinary people. However, heterosexuality remains the hegemonic gender norm in most societies that sidelines and discriminates homosexuals and individuals with diverse genders such as the LGBTQI. "All gender-diverse children, adolescents, and adults face challenges related to social and familial acceptance, and these challenges can lead to lasting mental health concerns" (Diamond 2020, 2). Stigmatization, victimization, and bullying are still the common experience of nonbinary and gender-diverse individuals, especially among young people (James et al., 2016).

Call to Inculturation and Adoption of Gender Diversity

Gender diversity and existence of gender-diverse people such as the LGBTQI are existing the world that require moral and apostolic recognition by the Catholic Church. Nonbinary Catholics can only be fully understood by actual immersion of Catholic leaders in their actual lives and struggles against discrimination. There is no substitute with personal encounters and dialogue between Catholic bishops and the LGBTQI Catholics. No amount of philosophizing can make Catholic bishops and moral theologians sympathetic to their personal plight and struggle of LGBTQI people and implement Pope Francis's synodal exhortation to love the marginalized, the voiceless, and those in the peripheries of the Church and society to realize his vision of a synodal church.

Shifting the philosophical approach founded on natural law theory and gender complementarity as theological and theoretical framework of the Catholic Church's moral teaching on sex and gender is indeed a call for inculturation, reexamining conceptual tools and update them in the light of Pope Francis's inductive theology to respond to the signs of the times. The social movement to recognize gender diversity and LGBTQI rights and inclusivity has been growing stronger in recent years. But the Catholic Church's basic philosophical and metaphysical theoretical moral on sex and gender could not accommodate contemporary gender theories, which are seen by the Vatican as "gender ideology."

Unless the Church's moral magisterium would shift its approach from philosophical to sociological and scientific on sex and gender diversity without abandoning the fundamental divine teaching that God created persons in his own image and likeness, inculturation would be a formidable task. Conversely speaking, St. Thomas Aquinas did not actually invent his philosophy and natural law theory for the good of the Church during his time. He adopted them from the pagan philosophy of Aristotle and Stoic concept of natural law and reframe them to inculturate or adapt the Christian message during the Medieval period, although several of their aspects are still relevant in today's world.

However, these adaptations by Aquinas are not absolute conceptual frameworks to always preach Christ's teachings throughout history. The philosophical approach to moral issues using natural law is not a "dogma" that is not subject to change, but only a cultural and conceptual tool to apply the

Catholic Church's moral principles in society when appropriate. This deductive philosophical approach could not cover all social and moral contingencies of gender and gender diversity in the contemporary world.

Therefore, the Catholic Church needs to explore the inductive and social science approach to update its teachings on sex, gender, and gender diversity. The main question for the full inclusion of the LGBTQI community in the Church is this: To what extent can the Church and Pope Francis compromise its basic moral framework based on natural law to embrace the scientific and inductive approach to sex and gender of sociologist, feminists, and LGBTQI activists to achieve inculturation and an inclusive synodal church, one that welcomes the marginalized and people with divergent views?

Resolving Gender Ideology as a Moral Panic

In the Catholic Church, the concept of moral panics has not been explored in understanding gender ideology, although it is utilized by some studies in Europe and some parts of Latin American countries. Catholic theologians and scholars have not been using the sociological concept of moral panics analyze the real nature of "gender ideology" as a form of exaggeration or moral panic. Investigating "gender ideology" as a form of moral panic in relation to Pope Francis's new synodal theological approach has escaped Catholic sociologists' attention.

There are some studies that characterized "gender ideology" as a moral panic. However, their focus tends to be particular and micro such as GI's impact on children's learning in the classroom (e.g., Da Silva Pereira 2023). No sociological studies that critically analyze gender ideology's alleged grave threats to society in the macro level, such as its dangers to humanity's survival, the moral foundation of the family, children's welfare, and human dignity, through the lens of Pope Francis's inductive synodal theology and sociology of gender and morality.

One important aspect of synodality is recognizing and respecting diversity of people's views and listening to marginalized persons in the Church and society. Sociologists, feminists, and gender activists are among the marginalized people in the Catholic Church. To welcome gender diverse and discriminated individuals in society in the Christian community, Francis's envisioned a synodal church to embrace all in the Church.

Despite his strong resistance to gender and gender ideology, Pope Francis's latest ecclesial reform project on synodality and inductive synodal theology encourages listening, consultation, and assimilation of the scientific methods in moral theologizing. Synodality promises a new inculturation process that incorporates the sociological and research findings on sex and gender in contemporary Catholic Church to resolve the conceptual conflict between the theological and sociological views on sexuality, gender, and gender diversity in the contemporary world.

Pope Francis's Inductive Synodal Theology and LGBTQI

In his inductive theological method, the Pope Francis insists that Catholic theology should begin with people's daily experiences in society before theologizing. This implies that understanding sex and gender should commence first with the social and cultural experiences of people in dealing with their gender identity. The open letter of a group of Catholic students, theologians, and ministers to Pope Francis and the Dicastery on the Doctrine of the Faith that protested the declaration of *Dignitas Infinita* [Infinite Dignity] for not considering the gender experience of transgenders and nonbinary people in charactering human dignity is an indication that the traditional deductive philosophical approach to gender is no longer adequate (National Catholic Register 2024). Scientific research has shown that people's biological sex assigned during birth may not necessarily reflect their gender identity and their personal expressions of masculinity and femininity in society.

Thus, the sociological realization that people's gender may not reflect their genitalia and biological make-up is empirically correct. The rise of transgender sexuality and the LGBTQI as distinct genders from heterosexuality is a social reality that the Catholic Church needs to recognize as the new call of the times. Transgenders are people whose "gender identity is different from their gender they were thought to be when they were born" (National Center for Transgender Equality 2023, para. 2). One main factor why transgender identity is rejected in society is the resistance of traditionists and conservatives of any same-sex relationship: "This is because neither male-male nor female-female relationships can fully embody the complementarity nature of humanity intended by God in creation" (Henegar 2011, 4). Transgenders and members of the LGBTQI could be categorized under the gender category of heterosexuality.

To Calib Day (2016), gender complementarianism based on the creation account is inappropriate trajectory to characterize the gender experience of gays and transgenders. In sociology, gender is socially and culturally conditioned.

"Human beings make other human beings into specific male and female genders" (Hopkins 2008, 576). The process of social learning and gender socialization determine people's gender identity and sexual orientation, which may not necessarily correspond to their biological sex.

A major obstacle toward a synodal understanding of sex and gender that is open to the divergent views of people behind gender ideology such as sociologists and, feminists is the lack of social science training and gender awareness of many Catholic clerics and moral theologians. The dominance of scholastic philosophy and philosophical theology in priestly education and theological studies promote prescriptive rather than descriptive and scientific thinking. It hinders the appreciation of the Catholic leaders and moral guardians on the positive elements of sociology of gender and feminist gender studies for understanding the real moral intention of transgenders and nonbinary people gender in altering their sex and gender in today's postmodern world.

The lack of familiarity with the nature and scientific method of sociology and the social sciences regarding gender and gender fluidity in society breeds contempt, moral panic, and inaccurate labelling of gender theories as gender ideology. One important area that Pope Francis's inductive synodal approach is to sharpen the empirical thinking of clerics and moral theologians in order to accurately assess the evolving moral situations of gender in contemporary society. Culture and society had greatly changed since the Medieval period when St. Thomas Aquinas synthesized Aristotelian philosophy and Catholic theology and popularized the natural law morality in the Catholic Church.

In today's contemporary culture and global society, people, technology, and material things are undergoing constant change or growing "liquidity" (Bauman 2000; Ritzer and Dean 2015). Because of this, the Catholic Church's main concern becomes empirical, that is, how to accurately review the fast-evolving facts of moral cases before applying the Church's moral principles. Scholastic philosophy and theology, which are taught to Catholic clerics and moral theologians during clerical formation are normative disciplines that cannot provide social contexts and scientific assessment of complex moral issues such as gender, gender diversity, LGBTQI inclusivity, and gender ideology in the contemporary age.

Thus, the time is ripe with Francis's synodality and inductive theology for the Catholic Church to shift its moral framework from deductive philosophical moral framework founded on natural law theory to an inductive sociological moral framework that utilizes the social science and feminist research and perspectives on sex and gender to fully understand transgenderism and the dynamics of gender in the contemporary world. Under this new and inculturated moral framework, living a homosexual and transgender life becomes more humane and morally acceptable as a distinct and legitimate gender lifestyle like heterosexuality in the Church and society. Gender ideology as a moral panic that threatens the binary understanding of humanity will fade and prepares the way for the full acceptance of the gender diverse members of LGBTQI community in the Catholic Church.

References

Ballano, Vivencio O. 2024. *Pope Francis's Synod on Synodality and Modern Sociology: Exploring the Synod's Behavioral and Research Aspects.* London: Routledge.

Corrêa, Sonia. 2017. "Gender Ideology: Tracking its Origins and Meanings in Current Gender Politics[6]." LSE (11 December 2017). https://blogs.lse.ac.uk/gender/2017/12/11/gender-ideology-tracking-its-origins-and-meanings-in-current-gender-politics/.

Deutsch, F.M. 2007. "Undoing Gender." *Gender Sociology.* 21(1): 106–127.

Diamond, Lisa M. 2020. "Gender Fluidity and Nonbinary Gender Identities Among Children and Adolescents." *Child Development Perspectives* 0(0):1-6: DOI: 10.1111/cdep.12366.

Fontanella, Lara, Maretti, Mara, and Sarra, Analinna. 2014. "Gender fluidity across the world: a Multilevel Item Response Theory approach." *Quality and Quantity* 48: 2553–2568 (2014). https://doi.org/10.1007/s11135-013-9907-4

Ford, Craig Jr. 2018. "Transgender Bodies, Catholic Schools, and a Queer Natural Law Theology of Exploration." *The Journal of Moral Theology* 7(1): 70-98.

Francis. 2016. "Meeting with the Polish Bishops: Address of His Holiness Pope Francis, 27 July 2016." Vatican: Dicastero per la Comunicazione—Libreria Editrice Vaticana https://www.vatican.va/content/francesco/en/speeches/2016/july/documents/papa-francesco_20160727_polonia-vescovi.html (accessed 30Aoril 2024).

---

6.   https://blogs.lse.ac.uk/gender/2017/12/11/gender-ideology-tracking-its-origins-and-meanings-in-current-gender-politics/

Graff, Agnieszka. 2016. "'Gender Ideology': Weak Concepts, Powerful Politics." *Religion and Gender* 6(2): 268-272. https://doi.org/10.18352/rg.10177.

Francis. 2016. "Meeting with the Polish Bishops: Address of His Holiness Pope Francis, 27 July 2016." Vatican: Dicastero per la Comunicazione—Libreria Editrice Vaticana https://www.vatican.va/content/francesco/en/speeches/2016/july/documents/papa-francesco_20160727_polonia-vescovi.html (accessed 30Aoril 2024).

James, S. E., Herman, J. L., Rankin, S., Keisling, M., Mottet, L., & Anafi,M. (2016).The report of the 2015 U.S. transgender survey. Washington, DC. Retrieved from https://www.transequality.org/site s/default/files/docs/USTS-Full-Report-FINAL.PDF

Mackay, Finn.2024. "'Gender Ideology' is All Around Us – But It's Not What the Tories Say It Is." *The Guardian* (19 January 2024). https://www.theguardian.com/commentisfree/2024/jan/19/gender-ideology-tories-ministers-schools-conservative.

Mares[7], Courtney. 2024. "Pope Francis: Gender Ideology is 'One of the Most Dangerous Ideological Colonizations' Today." *Catholic News Agency* (March 11, 2023). https://www.catholicnewsagency.com/news/253845/pope-francis-gender-ideology-is-one-of-the-most-dangerous-ideological-colonizations-today

Paternotte, David, and Kuhar, Roman. 2017. "Chapter 1: "'Gender Ideology' in Movement: An Introduction."'" In Roman Kuhar and David Paternotte, eds, *Anti-gender campaigns in Europe: Mobilizing Against Equality,* 1– 22. New York, London: Rowman & Littlefield International.

Philips, S.U. 2001. "Gender Ideology: Cross-Cultural Aspects." In Smelser, N.J. and Baltes, P.B. (eds) *International Encyclopedia of the Social & Behavioral Sciences,* pp. 1320–1344. Amsterdam, New York: Elsevier,

Red, Graeme. 2018. "The Buzzword: Fighting the 'Gender Ideology' Myth." *Human Rights Watch* (10 December 2018). https://www.hrw.org/news/2018/12/10/breaking-buzzword-fighting-gender-ideology-myth.

Scott, J.W. 1999. *Gender and the Politics of History.* Columbia University Press, New York.

Sheldon JP, Pfeffer CA, Jayaratne TE, Feldbaum M, and Petty EM. 2007. "Beliefs About the Etiology of Homosexuality and About the Ramifications

---

7.   https://www.catholicnewsagency.com/author/421/courtney-mares

of Discovering its Possible Genetic Origin. *Journal of Homosexuality* 52(3-4):111-50. https://doi.org/10.1300/J082v52n03_06. PMID: 17594974; PMCID: PMC4545255.

Vaggione, Jun Marco. 2020. "The Conservative Uses of Law: The Catholic Mobilization Against Gender Ideology" *Social Compass* 2020 67(2) 252–266. https://doi.org/10.1177/0037768620907561   journals.sagepub.com/home/scp.

Hammack-Aviran, C., Eilmus, A., Diehl, C., Gottlieb, K. G., Gonzales, G., Davis, L. K., and Clayton, E. W. 2022. LGBTQ+ Perspectives on Conducting Genomic Research on Sexual Orientation and Gender Identity. *Behavior Genetics* 52(4-5): 246–267. https://doi.org/10.1007/s10519-022-10105-y.

West, C., and Zimmerman, D.H. 1987. "Doing Gender." *Gender Sociology* 1(2): 125–151.

Zengarini, Lisa. 2024. "Pope Francis: Gender Ideology is the Ugliest Danger of Our Time." *Vatican News* (March 1, 2024). https://www.vaticannews.va/en/pope/news/2024-03/pope-francis-gender-ideology-is-the-ugliest-danger-of-our-time.html

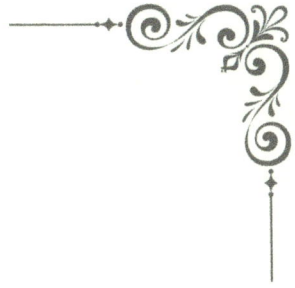

Chapter 4

LGBTQI Exclusion, Synodality, and the Morality of Sex Change; A Sociological Analysis

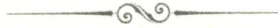

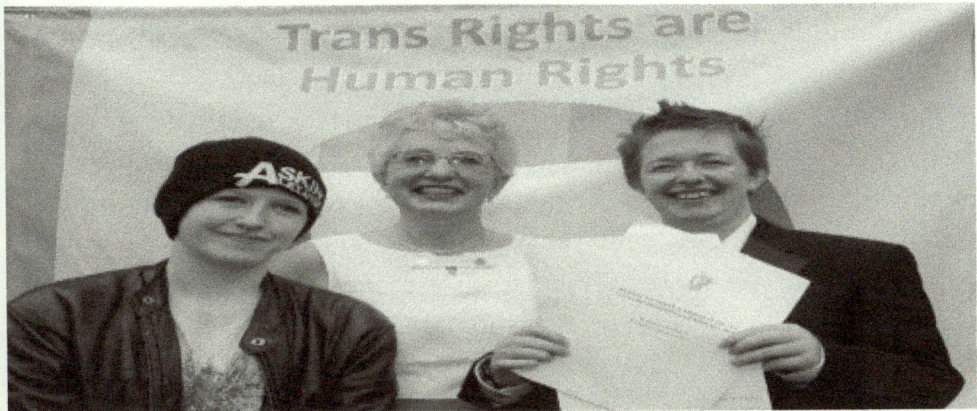

Photo: senator_katherine_zappone_young.jpg **Credit:** Flickr/Free-Images.com

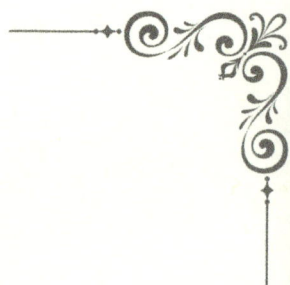

Introduction

Pope Francis is the first Catholic pope to show great compassion for members of the LGBTQI in contemporary times. In an interview with Associated Press, he criticized laws that criminalize homosexuality as unjust and declared that God loves all his children just as they are and called on Catholic bishops who support the repressive anti-homosexual laws to welcome lesbian, gay, bisexual, transgender, queer, and intersexual (LGBTQI) individuals into their dioceses or local churches (Winfield 2023). To Francis, homosexuality is not a crime.

To concretize his concern for the LGBQI, Francis approved the Vatican declaration *Dignitas Infinita* [Infinite Dignity] that condemned the criminalization of homosexuality in more than 70 countries and encourage of other faith leaders from around the globe to do the same. He also encouraged Catholic parents of queer children to love their children [1] and condemned parents who exclude them from their homes (Knox 2023). Francis attributed discriminatory attitudes against gays to cultural backgrounds and exhort his fellow bishops to undergo a process of conversion to recognize the dignity of everyone, including those with nonbinary sexuality and gender identity.

To date, Pope Francis's most aggressive action to assert the rights of the members of the LGBTQI group and welcome them in the Catholic Church is his approval of the document *Fiducia Supplicans* [On the Pastoral Meaning of Blessing] (FS), a declaration released by the Dicastery of Doctrine of the Faith, the doctrinal watchdog of the Vatican, that allowed the pastoral blessing of same-sex couples by Catholic priests as well as permitting adult transgenders to act as godparents in baptism (DDF 2023). Despite the stiff opposition of

---

1.   https://glaad.org/releases/pope-francis-compels-other-global-faith-leaders-reaffirm-laws-criminalizing-lgbtq-people/

conservative bishops, priests, and Catholics, Francis stood his ground, declaring that God welcomes all in the Church regardless of their sexual orientation. He made headlines when he declared in a media interview: "If a person is gay and seeks God and has good will, who am I to judge?" (BBC 2013).

Although the Catholic Church and Pope Francis have issued some pronouncements favoring homosexuality, homosexual union, and LGBTQI inclusion in the Church, no specific set of ecclesial teachings have been released thus far on transgender sexuality of Catholics as well as those who undergone sex change to align their biological sex to their gender orientation. As Craig Ford Jr. claims:

> At present, there is no official Catholic document that engages transgender persons directly as its principal subject. The result is that a determination about what exactly counts as "official church teaching" on the matter is complex, since any answer will essentially involve a collation of teachings, comments, and resources put out by the magisterium—more or less in passing—while focusing on other matters (Ford Jr. 2018, 75).

Official church documents that specifically provide moral guidelines on the ministry and pastoral care of transgender Catholics and members of the LGBTQI community in the Catholic Church are scarce and vague (Ford 2018; Canales 2016; Herriot and Callaghan 2019). Documents that deal with transgender sexuality and gender identity in the Church are usually done in passing and part of a larger conversations that are focused on family life, Catholic youth, and the environment (Roy-Steier 2021).

Pope Francis has issued some statements on transgender sexuality and the LGBTQI community. But these statements only reflect the traditional stance of the Catholic Church on sex and gender. In his comments relating to transgender persons in his encyclical *Laudato Si'* (2015) and apostolic exhortation *Amoris Laetitia* (2016), for instance, Francis reiterated the Magisterial teaching on sex and gender as "inseparably linked aspects of a singular reality and human identities as immutable and created by God" (Roy-Steier 2021, 3).

Like his predecessors Pope John Paul II and Pope Benedict XVI, Francis clearly upheld the traditional moral teaching that sees the metaphysical inseparability between sex and gender. He also condemned feminists, activists, and social scientists who oppose this teaching as people who advocate "gender ideology." As Craig Ford Jr. (2018, 77) contends:

> Francis gathers all opposition to current magisterial teaching with respect to sex and gender and gives it the name of 'ideology.' To do this, he creates a dichotomy between those who believe the truth, which is coextensive with the magisterium's position, and those who do not so believe the truth, who choose instead to give in to 'ideology.'

Objectives and Major Parts

The hot moral issues on gender, LGBTQI exclusion in society and in the Catholic Church, and sex change by transgender Catholics are complicated cases. It requires an accurate sociological understanding of the societal context why they continue to persist in society and in the Church. This chapter primarily attempts to firs distinguish the old deductive philosophical approach to Catholic morality and Pope Francis's inductive synodal approach to theological and moral issues. snodalanalyze the morality of sex change among transgender people in the Catholic Church, applying the synodal approach and inductive theological method of Pope Francis and some tenets of the sociology of morality.

It intends to first analyze inductively the moral situation and societal context of sex change in today's contemporary world using the current sociological and social science research and literature before applying the Church's moral principles and making resolution on how the Catholic Church should deal guide Catholics on sex change and transgender sexuality.

This chapter has three parts. The first part provides the theoretical framework of this study that distinguishes the current philosophical approach to moral issues such as sexuality and gender that applies the natural law theory and the inductive synodal method of Pope Francis and the sociological approach to gender and morality. It argues that the inductive synodal theological approach and modern sociological method are adequate tools to understand transgender sexuality and sex change among Catholics to enhance the inclusivity of the LGBTQI group in the Catholic Church.

The second part broadly investigates the societal and ecclesial contexts of the LGBTQI exclusion and harassment and why transgenders seek gender enhancement and sex change. It clarifies the current personal struggles and social harassment of transgenders in school, church, and immediate social environment, aiming to understand their motive for gender enhancement treatment and sex change.

The last part critically analyzes the morality of gender treatment and sex change applying the inductive sociological-synodal approach rather than the deductive philosophical moral approach based on natural law. It also attempts to analyze the Catholic morality of sex change using the principle of double effect.

Overall, it contends that Pope Francis's inductive synodal approach and sociological method can guide the Catholic Church for dealing with sexuality and gender diversity of the LGBTQI Catholics for the inclusion of transgenders in the Catholic Church. It also contends that the motive of transgenders is of primary importance in judging their moral decision for sex change. Judging the external act of sex change using the natural law moral framework is inadequate without first knowing the motive and lived experiences of transgenders in the Church and society as demanded by Pope Francis's inductive synodal theology.

Theoretical Framework
Deductive Moral Approach
The traditional church teaching that is based on the Thomistic natural law theory opposes all forms of homosexuality as intrinsically disordered not because it primarily violates biological laws but because it contravenes the logic of natural law theory that sees sex and gender as ahistorical and immutable and that only heterosexuality and gender complementarity are the fundamental norms for being a "natural" and normal person in the Catholic Church.

Pope John Paul II (1998) in his *Fides et Ratio* [Faith and Reason, #83), for example, argues for a need of a philosophical and metaphysical method in Catholic morality. He contends for "the need of a philosophy of genuinely metaphysical range, capable, that is, of transcending empirical data in order to attain something absolute, ultimate and foundational in its search for truth... for adequate understanding of the moral good" (Long 2013, 110). To St. Thomas, law is a thing of reason or intellect. In his many writings, he expounds an intellectualist account of law that influenced Catholic tradition:

> According to this tradition...the received law is nothing less than our human participation in the eternal law, the divine mind disposing all

created things to their ends. Human law, therefore, far from being the arbitrary result of agreement and command, receives its warrant from its being derived from the natural law, our sharing in the divine providential governance of the universe. (Brennan 2010, 2)

The inseparability of sex and gender based on natural law entered Catholic sexual teaching recently as a concept during the pontificate of John Paul II, especially as he developed it in his collections of homilies that became known as the Theology of the Body. "Masculinity and femininity express the twofold aspect of man's somatic constitution...This meaning, one can say, consists in reciprocal enrichment." Refracting this theological perspective into the natural law tradition, this gender essentialism paired with gender complementarity is understood to be a natural complementarity between the genders" (Ford 2018, 81).

Because of this influential theology espoused by Pope John Paul II and reaffirmed by Pope Benedict XVI and Pope Francis, the Catholic Church has inappropriately and indiscriminately categorized all views and explanations that oppose this theology and official sexual teachings of the Magisterium, including the inductive scientific approaches of the social sciences as "gender ideology" (Ford Jr. 2018). This labelling does acknowledge, however, the basic difference in perspective and method between the traditional Catholic morality and the social sciences. The current Catholic moral theology sees the inseparability between sex and gender while sociology and the social sciences view sex as biological and gender as social and cultural.

Furthermore, the Compendium of the Social Doctrine of the Church (CSDC) (Pontifical Council for Justice and Peace, 2005, #224) "Faced with theories that consider gender identity as merely the cultural and social product of the interaction between the community and the individual, independent of personal sexual identity without any reference to the true meaning of sexuality" still insists on gender complementarity and heteronormativity:

Everyone, man and woman, should acknowledge and accept his sexual identity. Physical, moral, and spiritual difference and complementarities are oriented towards the goods of marriage and the flourishing of family life...' According to this perspective, it is obligatory that positive law be conformed to the natural law, according to which sexual identity is indispensable, because it is the objective condition for forming a couple in marriage. (Pontifical Council for Justice and Peace, 2005, #224)

The deductive and philosophical approach in resolving the moral issues on transgender sexuality and inclusivity of the LGBTQI Catholics in the Catholic Church theoretically from afar does not generate Christian sympathy, Christian love, and genuine concern for transgender Catholics. It merely judges the external acts of transgenders from a set of metaphysical norms based on Thomistic natural law theory and scholastic philosophy as deviant and "unnatural" without knowing first the real situation of the LGBTQI Catholics in the peripheries of the Catholic Church. This is precisely what Pope Francis, the pope of the peripheries wanted to be changed in his synodality and inductive synodal theology.

Sociology of Gender and Inductive Synodal Approach

Sociology and the social sciences generally oppose this ontological inseparability of sex and gender based on religious criteria. To social scientists, sex is biological and in-born, determined by the person's genitalia, while gender is social and cultural in nature, learned by the individual and conditioned by his or her socialization in society and local culture. Seeing sex and gender as one and immutable is largely an influence of a purely philosophical approach that predominantly applies the Thomistic natural law theory and deductive reasoning that disregards people's lived experiences in society.

Lacking in sociology and social science education in clerical training as well as active dialogue between Catholic theologians and sociologists, it is understandable that clerics and Catholic hierarchy still rely on natural law theory, philosophy, and reasoning in doing moral theology and deciding moral cases deductively. St. Thomas Aquinas popularized the natural law theory in Catholic moral theology that utilized a philosophical method to resolve moral cases in the Catholic Church. He made the most influential formulation of this theory in the 13th century, which became central to the moral magisterium of the Catholic Church (Long 2013).

"Natural law tradition continued to be preserved and developed by Roman Catholic moral theologians, with the results that it came to be associated with

Catholic thought—an association that persists to this day" (Porter 2005, 32-33). However, Pope Francis has been introducing welcome reforms to the RCC that prioritize human experience and inductive approach as the starting point to resolve moral issues such as transgender sexuality and the LGBTQI inclusivity in the RCC. In the light of his latest actions and pronouncements in *Fiducia Supplicans* [Supplicating Trust] and *Ad Theologiam Promovendam* [To Promote Theology] (APT), more can be expected from Francis to reform Catholic moral theology.

Pope Francis's ecclesial reform process called synodality and synodal theology encourage moral theologians to resolve ethical and ecclesial issues inductively and appreciate the contribution of sociological and social science approaches in ethical cases. As Ford Jr. (2018) contends, Because Catholic tradition holds that both faith and reason come from God and work together to reveal truth, empirical evidence and theoretical knowledge can be used to help inform morality and guide pastoral practice. "The Magisterium has not shied away from utilizing sociological research and scientific data to inform its positions, teachings, and responses to various social, political, cultural, and religious issues" (Roy-Steier 2021, 1).

Francis's emphasizes on listening and consultation with people before making moral and doctrinal judgments in his synodality. The declaration on blessing of homosexual couples in *Fiducia Supplicans* and the paradigm shift in doing Catholic theology in *Ad Theogiam Promovendam* clearly tend to sidestep the deductive philosophical approach to morality based on natural law. Francis is insisting that understanding first the human experience is necessary before theological reflection and moral decision.

Thus, one can expect that Francis would improve the Catholic Church's moral stance towards homosexuality, transgender sexuality, and the LGBTQI inclusivity in the future, one that is more sympathetic to the personal difficulties of transgender Catholics and more open to empirical, inductive, and sociological methods to achieve a synodal church that fully welcomes the marginalized LGBTQI in the Christian community.

The Catholic Church's application of moral principles is not infallible and may be subjected to change and inculturation, depending on the Magisterium's accurate reading or appreciation of moral situations. The sudden shift of allowing blessing to homosexual couples instead of prohibiting it in earlier pronouncement by the Vatican indicates that moral teachings in the Church can change in time.

Catholic moral theologians should go down from their pedestals and immerse with the poor, the marginalized, and ordinary people in the Church and understand their innermost thoughts and concerns. To Pope Francis, Catholic theologians should "smell like their sheep". Life is bigger than their theories and ideas.

Discrimination of Transgenders in Society and Catholic Church

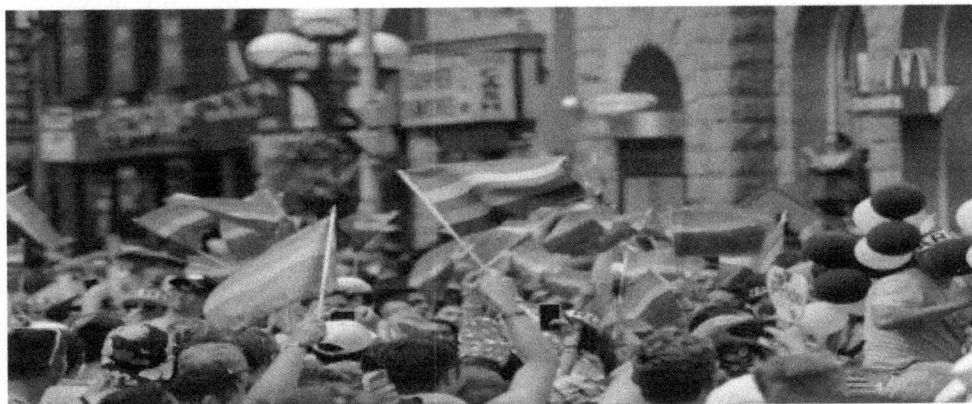

Photo: gay_gay_pride_pride.jpg **Credit:** Pixabay/Free-Images.com

"Public awareness and the visibility of transgender and gender-variant individuals has increased in recent times, with a significant rise in public discussions concerning transgender issues over the last decade (e.g., improving legal rights, access to healthcare, gender-neutral bathrooms, etc.; Bockting et al., 2016; Stroumsa, 2014). Yet despite increased awareness, transgender people remain subject to significant discrimination and harassment (Lombardi, 2009; Miller & Grollman, 2015; Stotzer, 2008). A growing body of evidence indicates that a majority of transgender people have been assaulted due to their gender identify (Campbell, Hinton, and Anderson 2019, 21).

"Unfortunately, many Christian faith communities perpetuate discriminatory stances, leaving transgender people without a spiritual home (Bockting and Cesaretti, 2001). Findings from 27,715 participants in the 2015 U.S. Transgender Survey indicated that nearly one in five (19%) of respondents who had ever been part of a spiritual or religious community left due to rejection and 39% left out of fear of being rejected because they were transgender (James et al., 2016). Discrimination and negative responses toward diverse gender identities from members of religious communities contribute to weakened ties to formal religious institutions (Bockting, Knudson, & Goldberg, 2006). Further, leaving transgender people without a welcoming place of worship can contribute to the rejection of religion altogether" (Benson, Westerfield, and van Eeden-Moorefield 2018, 396-397).

"Research clearly demonstrates that transgender people in the U.S. encounter significant ignorance and discrimination in many aspects of their lives, including family rejection, housing, and employment discrimination, and access to healthcare" (Benson, Westerfield, and van Eeden-Moorefield 2018, 396). Anecdotal evidence shows tremendous rejection of transgenders in the Church and society and moral pressures from the Catholic Church to conform to heteronormativity despite their homosexual orientation and identity.

One transgender student named Leelah, for instance, committed suicide by walking onto a highway to end her suffering and discrimination. She left a note before her death to illustrate the struggles of transgenders in life:

> After a summer of having almost no friends plus the weight of having to think about college, save money for moving out, keep my grades up, go to church each week and feel like shit because everyone there is against everything I live for, I have decided I've had enough. I'm never going to transition successfully, even when I move out. I'm never going to be happy with the way I look or sound. I'm never going to have enough friends to satisfy me. I'm never going to have enough love to satisfy me. I'm never going to find a man who loves me. I'm never going to be happy. Either I live the rest of my life as a lonely man who wishes he were a woman, or I live my life as a lonelier woman who hates herself. There's no winning. There's no way out. I'm sad enough already, I don't need my life to get any worse. People say "it gets better" but that isn't true in my case. It gets worse. Each day I get worse.[1] (Ford Jr.2018, 70).

National surveys, population studies, and demographic analyses monitoring the economic security, health, safety, and well-being of gender and sexual minorities continue to report that transgender people remain one of the most marginalized, at-risk, and disenfranchised populations within the United States (Badgett et al. 2019; Hunter et al. 2018; James et al. 2016; CAP & MAP 2015; and Grant et al. 2011). Because of discrimination and marginalization, research suggests that attempted suicide is disproportionally higher among the transgender populations (Blosnich et. al. 2013).

In the Catholic Church, transgender Catholics are among the ostracized members of the Christian community. Several dioceses of the RCC in the United States, for instance, have released documents about transgender people in the Church but most of these documents focuses only on the literal interpretation of the Genesis story about the gender complementarity between male and female and has not recognized the lived experiences and personal struggles of real Catholic transgenders and members of the LGBTQI group. They have not acknowledged the dignity of transgender Catholics. They also ignore the social sciences' evolving view on gender, failing to provide the appropriate pastoral care to transgender members in their dioceses (Kuzma 2023).

An early study in the United States (US) showed that between 4 and 5 per one hundred thousand persons are transgenders (Blosnich et. al. 2013). An American Hospital Survey (2013) also revealed that Catholic health care services across the US saw more than 5.2 million persons per year, which imply that these hospitals will care more than 200 transpersons annually. This figure did not include Catholic transgenders in other countries. Despite the growing number of transgenders in the Church, conservative Catholic bishops continue to deny their existence and still insist on heterosexuality as the only norm to be "natural" and normal human beings in the Catholic Church.

To practice their Christian faith, transgender Catholics therefore are forced to face rejection in the Christian community and coercion to conform to the Catholic Church's heteronormativity. They also experience rebukes from fellow Catholics and several bishops. In the Archdiocese of Milwaukee, for example, church personnel are barred to use transgenders' preferred pronouns that reflect their gender identity, a policy that aims to object trans-supportive "gender theory." It states that "all interactions and policies, parishes, organizations, and institutions are to recognize only a person's biological sex" (Crary 2022, para. 4).

The diocese of Marquette also seems to discriminate the LGBTQI Catholics with the issuance of new anti-transgender policy in the local church, requiring all people in parishes, schools, and other Catholic organizations in the archdiocese to use bathrooms appropriate to their sex and observe heterosexual dress code. It also instructs parish pastors to deny LGBTQI parishioners the sacraments of baptism as well as receiving holy communion during the Mass unless they repent and return to heterosexuality, a new policy that was signed itself by the local bishop (Crary 2022).

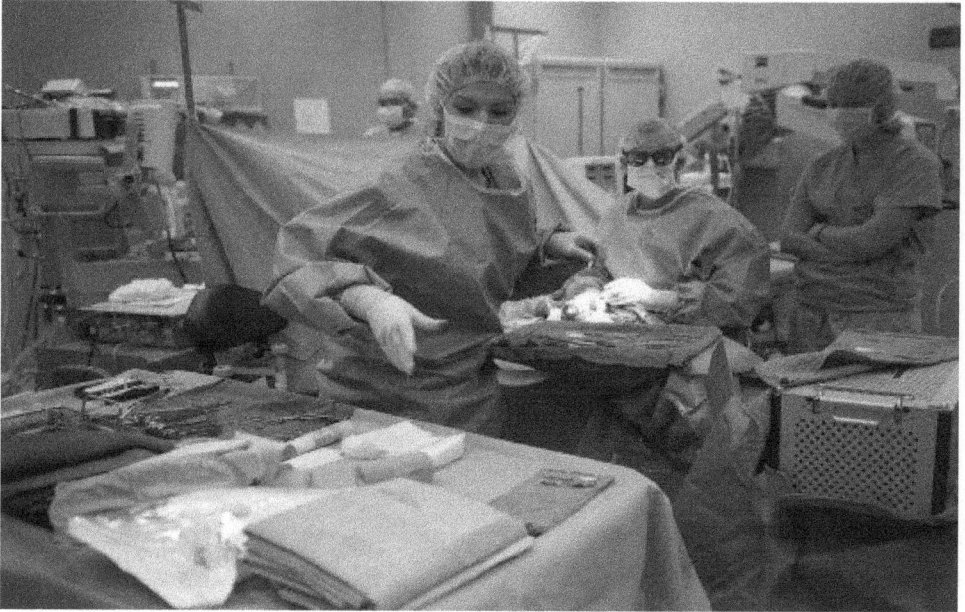

Photo: medicine_medical_surgery_nurse.jpg Credit: pixabay/Free-Images.com

Owing to the advancement of medical technology and transgender surgery, more and more Catholics are changing their biological sex to suit their gender and sexual orientation. Despite this fact, the Catholic Church remains distant and indifferent to the real struggles and discrimination experienced by transgender Catholics. It still formulates moral guidelines on sex and gender based on the deductive philosophical approach and Thomistic natural law theory rather on scientific research based on the real experiences of transgender Catholics.

Because of the lack of scientific sensitivity and gender awareness training, several bishops and priests continue to view homosexuality and transgender sexuality as "unnatural" and deviation from normal human maturity using the deductive philosophical approach of Thomistic natural law theory. Instead of listening and entering the lives of real transgenders and LGBTQI group in the Church as envisioned by Pope Francis in his inductive synodal theology, proponents of the deductive philosophical method only formulate judgment against transgenders using logic and reasoning without immersing first into the real world of the LGBTQI.

Thus, Pope Francis encourages bishops "to nurture a culture of listening that transcends daily tasks and positions, giving value to relationships and maintaining an evangelical spirit marked by the ability to listen sincerely and without judgment" (Bordoni 2023, para. 8). This synodal listening includes empathizing with homosexuals and the LGBTQI who have long been ostracized silently in the Church because of homophobia and heteronormativity that only accept heterosexuals as morally normal persons in the Catholic Church.

The Morality of Sex Change and Principle of Double Effect

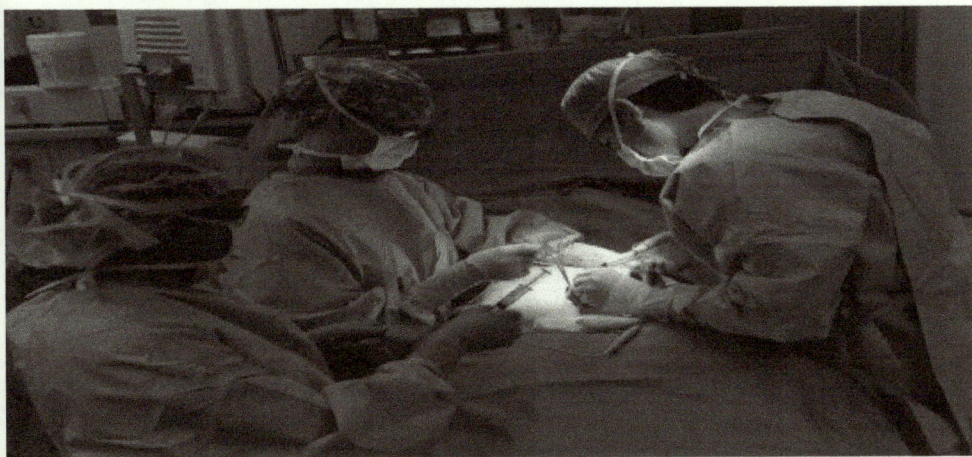

Photo: surgery_surgeons_operation_medical_2.jpg **Credit:** Pixabay/Free-Images.com

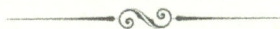

Applying a synodal, inductive, and sociological approach to Catholic morality implies investigating first the real intentions of people and the empirical reality before theologizing and moral judgment. This approach is consistent with the traditional See-Judge-Act methodology with "seeing" or accurately knowing the moral situation as the starting point of moral analysis and the traditional moral approach in judging morality. In applying the application of the Catholic

Church's Catholic social teaching, understanding the empirical reality should be prioritized to appropriately apply the moral principles and come up with an adequate action.

In evaluating the sources of morality in the Catholic Church, the Catechism of the Catholic Church (1993, #1750) highlights the following components: the object chosen, the end in view or the intention, and the circumstance of the action. Thus, the intention or motive of the actor in an act is crucial to evaluate morality:

> 1752 In contrast to the object, the intention resides in the acting subject. Because it lies at the voluntary source of an action and determines it by its end, intention is an element essential to the moral evaluation of an action. The end is the first goal of the intention and indicates the purpose pursued in the action. The intention is a movement of the will toward the end: it is concerned with the goal of the activity. It aims at the good anticipated from the action undertaken.

Understanding human intention and not just the external act to understand the morality of an action is in consonance with Max Weber's sociological concept on verstehen or understanding motives together with the person's external action or stereotype to fully understand the meaning of his or her act. This implies putting oneself into the shoes of the other in order to fully understand his or her behavior. This also requires—what Pope Francis always insists in his synodality—listening to people's concerns before passing theological or moral judgment.

Passing moral judgment based on appearance and external actions of transgenders without first listening and knowing their true intentions or motives on why they behave differently from heterosexuality and undergo sex change is inadequate. Members of the LGBTQI are personally struggling on how to reconcile their sex and gender identity. As Canner et al. (2028, 609) contends:

> "Transgender individuals have a gender identity that differs from their sex at the time of birth. To address this incongruence, many transgender patients may seek gender-affirming interventions to

achieve concordance between self-identified gender, physical appearance, and function. Gender-affirming interventions may include hormone therapy and gender-affirming surgical procedures such as genital or breast surgery and facial contouring" (Canner et al. 2018, 609).

"Transsexual persons that are attracted by individuals of the opposite biological sex are more likely to change sexual orientation. Qualitative reports suggest that the individual's biography, autogynephilic and autoandrophilic sexual arousal, confusion before and after transitioning, social and self-acceptance, as well as concept of sexual orientation itself may explain this phenomenon" (Auer et al. 2014, 1). A study by Zavlin et al (2018, 178), for instance, revealed that:

[p]atients rated their surgical satisfaction of most items with mean scores above 7 on a 0–10-point scale. Many items evaluating everyday life activities improved significantly after SRS compared to T0 ($p <$ 0.01). All but one patient (97.5%) reported no regrets about having undergone surgery, and the majority recommended it to other patients with gender dysphoria. Femininity and sexual activity increased significantly postoperatively ($p <$ 0.01). Satisfaction with intercourse and orgasm was high: 6.70 and 8.21, respectively, on a 0–10 scale.

Transgenders' intention to change sex is primarily not mere vanity but a desire for social acceptance, wholeness, and personal happiness. They intend to align their sex or biological make-up to their gender identity and sexual orientation. Plastic surgeons who performed sex change for transgenders reported satisfaction of patients as regards to the functional and sexual outcomes, revealing positive effects on their lives (Zavlin et al. (2018). They also revealed that "even minor surgical alterations in transgender patients can have a profound improvement on patients' self-esteem and functioning. These surgical procedures range from penile to neovaginal reconstruction, and chest wall contouring (Canner et al. 2018, 609).

Sex change can make people sterile, but one must judge its morality based on the transgender's intention, which is basically good, that is, to attain wholeness and compatibility between his or sex and gender. The traditional tool of moral analysis in the Catholic Church called the "principle of double effect" to judge a complex act with two effects: one is good, and the other is bad is appropriate to analyze the Catholic morality of sex change. As Dr. Carol Bayley (2016, 3) contends:

> This tool allows us to think through whether a negative outcome is morally permissible when it is foreseen but not intended. The action undertaken must be good or at least neutral; the desired effect must be good; the bad effect must not be the means to the good effect and the action undertaken must be proportionate to the desired good outcome" (Bayley 2016, 3).

Using the moral principle of double effect, Dr. Carol Bayley (2016) then morally justifies sex change to suit the person's gender. She explains the unforeseen effect of sterility in sex change for transgenders. But the act of surgery is morally neutral. And the ultimate intention or motive of the intended effect is not evil but good:

> In the case of bottom surgery that will sterilize the person, I believe that we can use the rule of double effect in a similar way. The surgery itself is neutral. The good effect, from the perspective of the person undergoing it, is that his or her body will come to present to the world the person in the gender he or she experiences inside. The relief of suffering this represents is profound. (Bayley 2016, 4)

Sex change does not only provide personal satisfaction for transgenders but also legal recognition of changing their gender and name. Most current legal systems, like the Catholic Church, only recognizes heterosexuality and sex as the basis for gender. "Courts generally will not recognize a transgender person's chosen sex or gender without the undergoing sex change surgery, and preoperative transgender individuals are sometimes precluded from legal name change as well" (Ben-Asher 2006, 55). Transgenders can then enjoy legal status and other societal benefits if their gender is aligned with their sex.

The crux of the issue of why the Catholic Church still rejects transgender sexuality and identity as well as sex change is the traditional belief based on a metaphysical understanding that sex and gender are inseparable and immutable, thus upholding heterosexuality as the only norm for sexual and gender identity. This is contrary to the sociological and inductive approach that first investigate the empirical reality and real intention and motive of the person in judging transgender sexuality and identity.

Clearly, sex is biological, but gender is social and experiential, learned by the person through the normal socialization process in society. Gender is not a personal intention, but a social product not primarily intended by the person. Thus, it is not a sign of immaturity on the part of the person, as the traditional moral teaching of the Church still claims if he or she assumes a transgender sexuality and identity after birth.

"Gender" is a social behavior or norm while "sex" is permanent, nonnegotiable, and objective that is based on biology. While gender is often considered to be something that bodies *do*, sex is often considered what *are*" (Ben-Asher 2006, 52-53). "The words *heterosexual, homosexual* and *bisexual* describe sexual attraction, grounded in biology but affected by culture. Attraction can be fluid and changing, particularly in a culture that privileges heterosexual attraction as "normal" and homosexual or bisexual attraction as abnormal" (Bayley 2016, 2).

Conclusion

This chapter has analyzed the moral situation and empirical foundation of the emerging transgender sexuality in the contemporary world and how a synodal church as envisioned by Pope Francis in his innovative SoS can deal with transgenderism and LGBTQI inclusivity. Using Francis's inductive theology and the sociological perspective as the general conceptual framework, it has attempted to resolve the delicate moral situation of changing one's sex or biological make-up using the modern cosmetic technology to follow his or her gender orientation and sexual preference through the principle of double effect as well as through the lens of sociology and synodality.

It argued that the synodal and sociological approach can guide the Catholic Church on how to appropriately judge the sexuality and gender orientation of transgender Catholics beyond appearance and external acts and examine real personal struggles and personal motives on why they resort to gender enhancement and sex change for greater social acceptance and inclusivity in the Church and society. This chapter recommends a regular and synodal consultations between Catholic bishops and transgender Catholics and members of the LGBTQI group both in the diocesan level during Synod on Synodality's churchwide consultations and roundtable discussions during the general assembly in Rome.

References

Abend, Gabriel. 2010. "What's New and What's Old about the New Sociology of Morality." Pp. 561–86 in Handbook of the Sociology of Morality, edited by S. Hitlin and S. Vaisey. New York: Springer.

Arrupe, Fr. Pedro S.J. 1978. ""On Inculturation, to the Whole Society." *Portal to Jesuit Studies Website*. https://jesuitportal.bc.edu/research/documents/ 1978_arrupeinculturationsociety/#:~:text=With%20the%20letter%2C%20issued 2

Auer, Matthias K., Fuss, Johannes, Hohne, Nina, Stalla, Gunter K., Sievers, Caroline. 2014. "Transgender Transitioning and Change of Self-Reported Sexual Orientation." *PLoS ONE* 9(10): e110016. https://doi.org/10.1371/ journal.pone.0110016.

Bayley, Carol. 2016. "Transgender Persons and Catholic Healthcare." *Healthcare Ethics USA* 24(1): 1-17.

BBC News. 2013. "Pope Francis: Who Am I to Judge Gay People?" *BBC News Website* (July 29, 2013). https://www.bbc.com/news/ world-europe-23489702.

---

2.   https://jesuitportal.bc.edu/research/documents/

1978_arrupeinculturationsociety/#_853ae90f0351324bd73ea615e6487517__4c761f170e016836ff8449820

2b99827__853ae90f0351324bd73ea615e6487517_text_43ec3e5dee6e706af7766fffea512721_With_0bcef9

c45bd8a48eda1b26eb0c61c869_20the_0bcef9c45bd8a48eda1b26eb0c61c869_20letter_0bcef9c45bd8a48ed

a1b26eb0c61c869_2C_0bcef9c45bd8a48eda1b26eb0c61c869_20issued_0bcef9c45bd8a48eda1b26eb0c61c

869_20on_c0cb5f0fcf239ab3d9c1fcd31fff1efc_the_0bcef9c45bd8a48eda1b26eb0c61c869_20local_0bcef9c

45bd8a48eda1b26eb0c61c869_20Church_0bcef9c45bd8a48eda1b26eb0c61c869_20and_0bcef9c45bd8a48

eda1b26eb0c61c869_20to

Ben-Asher, Noa. 2006. "The Necessity of Sex Change: A Struggle for Intersex and Transsex Liberties." 29 *Harvard Journal of Law & Gender* 51 (2006), http://digitalcommons.pace.edu/lawfaculty/591/.

Benson, Kristen; Westerfield, Eli; and van Eeden-Moorefield, Bradley, "Transgender People's Reflections on Identity, Faith, and Christian Faith Communities in the U.S." 2018. Department of Family Science and Human Development Scholarship and Creative Works. 186. https://digitalcommons.montclair.edu/familysci-facpubs/186.

Blosnich, John R., Brown, George R., Shipherd, Jillian C. Kauth, Michael, Piegari, Rebecca I., and Bossarte. Robert M. 2013. "Prevalence of Gender Identity Disorder and Suicide Risk Among Transgender Veterans Utilizing Veterans Health Administration Care." *American Journal of Public Health*: October 2013, Vol. 103, No. 10, pp. e27-e32.

Bordoni, Linda. 2023. "Pope Asks Journalists for Help to Communicate Synod." Vatican News (August 26, 2023). https://www.vaticannews.va/en/pope/news/2023-08/pope-francis-journalism-synod-synodality-truth-award-audience.html.

Brennan, Patrick McKinley. 2011. "Human Law and Natural Law in the Catholic Tradition: Authoritative Guides to the Good Life." In Piderit, John Jay, and Morey, Melanie May, eds, *Teaching the Tradition: A Disciplinary Approach to the Catholic Intellectual Tradition*. Oxford, UK: Oxford University Press.

Brickel, Chris. 2009. "Chapter 19: Sexuality, Morality and Society." In Byrnes, Giselle, ed, *The New Oxford History of New Zealand*. Auckland, NZ: Oxford University Press.

Campbell, Marianne, Hinton, Jordan D. X., and Anderson, Joel R. 2019. "A Systematic Review of the Relationship Between Religion and Attitudes Toward Transgender and Gender-Variant People." *International Journal of Transgenderism* 20(1): 21-38. https://doi.org/10.1080/15532739.2018.1545149.

Canner JK, Harfouch O, Kodadek LM, Pelaez D, Coon D, Offodile AC 2nd, Haider AH, Lau BD. Temporal Trends in Gender-Affirming Surgery Among Transgender Patients in the United States. JAMA Surg. 2018 Jul 1;153(7):609-616. doi: 10.1001/jamasurg.2017.6231. PMID: 29490365; PMCID: PMC5875299.

Catechism of the Catholic Church. 1993. Libreria Editrice Vaticana. https://www.vatican.va/arc hive/ENG0015/_INDEX.HTM#fonte.

Crary, David. 2022. "Rejection or Welcome: Transgender Catholics Encounter Both." *AP News Website* (February 26, 2022. https://apnews.com/article/lifestyle-religion-united-states-gender-identity-marquette-368a622737d78df1f1f254a1e8e68aaf.

DDF (Dicastery of the Doctrine of the Faith). 2023. "On the Pastoral Meaning of Blessings." Vatican: The Roman Curia. Available at: https://www.vatican.va/roman_curia/congregations/cfaith/documents/rc_ddf_doc_20231218_fiducia-supplicans_en.html.

Ford, Craig Jr. 2018. "Transgender Bodies, Catholic Schools, and a Queer Natural Law Theology of Exploration." *The Journal of Moral Theology* 7(1): 70-98.

Hitlin. Steven, and Vaisey, Stephen. 2013, eds, 2013. "Chapter 1: Back to the Future: Reviving the sociology of Morality." *The Sociology of Morality*. New York: Springer.

Hitlin, Steven and Vaisey, Stephen. 2013. "The New Sociology of Morality[3]." *Annual Review of Sociology* 2013 39 (1): 51-68.

Knox, Dallas. 2023. "Pope Francis Calls for the Inclusion of Trans People in Catholic Church Practices." *Glaad Website* (November 9, 2023). https://glaad.org/pope-francis-calls-for-the-inclusion-of-trans-people-in-catholic-practices/.

Kuzma, Maxwell. 2023. "Trans Catholics exist, and we deserve to participate in church life." *The National Catholic Reporter* (November 10, 2023). https://www.ncronline.org/opinion/guest-voices/trans-catholics-exist-and-we-deserve-participate-church-life.

Long, Steven A.2013. "Fundamental Errors of the New Natural Law Theory." The National Catholic Bioethics Quarterly[4] 13(1): 105-131. https://doi.org/10.5840/ncbq201313173.

Meier, S.C, Pardo, S.T., Labuski, C, and Babcock, J. 2013. Measures of Clinical Health among Female-to-Male Transgender Persons as a Function of Sexual Orientation. Arch Sex Behavior 42: 463–474.

---

3.   https://www.annualreviews.org/doi/abs/10.1146/annurev-soc-071312-145628

4.   https://www.pdcnet.org/collection-anonymous/browse?fp=ncbq

National Center for Transgender Equality. 2023. "Understanding Transgender People: The Basics." *National Center for Transgender Equality Website* (January 27, 2023). https://transequality.org/issues/resources/understanding-transgender-people-the-basics.

Pontifical Council for Justice and Peace, 2005. *Compendium of the Social Doctrine of the Church.* Vatican: Libreria Editrice Vaticana. https://www.vatican.va/roman_curia/pontifical_councils/justpeace/documents/rc_pc_justpeace_doc_20060526_compendio-dott-soc_en.html.

Pope Francis. 2013. *Evangelli Gaudium* [An Apostolic Exhortation on the Proclamation of the Gospel in Today's World]. Vatican: Dicastero per la Comunicazione - Libreria Editrice Vaticana. https://www.vatican.va/content/francesco/en/apost_exhortations/documents/papa-francesco_esortazione-ap_20131124_evangelii-gaudium.html.

Pope John Paul II. 1998. *Fides et Ratio* [Faith and Reason]: *An Encyclical on the Relationship Between Faith and Reason.* Vatican: Dicastero per la Comunicazione - Libreria Editrice Vaticana. https://www.vatican.va/content/john-paul-ii/en/encyclicals/documents/hf_jp-ii_enc_14091998_fides-et-ratio.html.

Roy-Steier, Stephanie. 2021. "Coming Up Short: The Catholic Church's Pastoral Response to the Transgender Crisis in America. *Religions* 12(337): 1-20. https://doi.org/10.3390/rel12050337

Stets, Jan E. and Carter, Michael J. 2012. "A Theory of the Self for the Sociology of Morality." *American Sociological Review* 77(1): 120–140.

The Associated Press. 2023. "Vatican moves closer to permitting transgender Catholics to be baptized." CBC (November 9, 2023). https://www.cbc.ca/news/world/vatican-pope-transgender-baptism-1.7023505.

Winfield, Nicole. 2023. "The AP Interview: Pope Says Homosexuality not a Crime." Associated Press (January 26, 2023). https://apnews.com/article/pope-francis-gay-rights-ap-interview-1359756ae22f27f87c1d4d6b9c8ce212.

Weber, Max. 2009. *From Max Weber: Essays in Sociology. First Edition.* London: Routledge.

Zavlin[5], Dmitry, Jürgen Schaff[6], Jean-Daniel Lellé[7], Kevin T. Jubbal[8], Peter Herschbach[9], Gerhard Henrich[10], Benjamin Ehrenberger[11], Laszlo Kovacs[12], Hans-Günther Machens[13] and Nikolaos A. Papadopulos[14].

[1] The acronym to collectively label nonbinary people or the third sex in society evolves in time. Some authors use the terms "LGBT" or "LGBTQ", while others apply the acronyms "LGBTQI", "LGBTQI+" or LGBTQIA+. More recent publications include "plus sign" (+) after the acronymto recognize the fluidity or evolving nature of gender. For brevity and consistency, this book uses "LGBTQI" throughout the text.

[2] Reach Out. n.d. "A teenager's story about coming out." para. 1.

[3] Reach Out. n.d. "A teenager's story about coming out." para. 1.

[4] New Ways Ministry. 2024. "What Transgender Catholics and Their Allies Are Saying About 'Dignitas Infinita.'" New Ways Ministry Website (10 April 2024), paras. 6-7. https://www.newwaysministry.org/2024/04/10/what-transgender-catholics-and-their-allies-are-saying-about-dignitas-infinita/

[5] National Catholic Reporter. 2024. "Catholic students, theologians, ministers write an open letter to Pope Francis." *National Catholic Reporter Website* (25 April 2024). https://www.ncronline.org/opinion/guest-voices/catholic-students-theologians-ministers-write-open-letter-pope-francis.

[6] Ibid., para. 15-15.

[7] "Just Let Us Be: Discrimination Against LGBT Students in the Philippines" 2017, para. 4.

---

5. https://link.springer.com/article/10.1007/s00266-017-1003-z#auth-Dmitry-Zavlin-Aff1-Aff2

6. https://link.springer.com/article/10.1007/s00266-017-1003-z#auth-J_rgen-Schaff-Aff3

7. https://link.springer.com/article/10.1007/s00266-017-1003-z#auth-Jean_Daniel-Lell_-Aff1

8. https://link.springer.com/article/10.1007/s00266-017-1003-z#auth-Kevin_T_-Jubbal-Aff4

9. https://link.springer.com/article/10.1007/s00266-017-1003-z#auth-Peter-Herschbach-Aff5

10. https://link.springer.com/article/10.1007/s00266-017-1003-z#auth-Gerhard-Henrich-Aff5

11. https://link.springer.com/article/10.1007/s00266-017-1003-z#auth-Benjamin-Ehrenberger-Aff1

12. https://link.springer.com/article/10.1007/s00266-017-1003-z#auth-Laszlo-Kovacs-Aff1

13. https://link.springer.com/article/10.1007/s00266-017-1003-z#auth-Hans_G_nther-Machens-Aff1

14. https://link.springer.com/article/10.1007/
s00266-017-1003-z#auth-Nikolaos_A_-Papadopulos-Aff1-Aff6

[8] Bishops Conference of England and Wales. 2024. "Bishops Issue Pastoral Reflection on Gender," paras. 1-3.

[9] The 2020 Trevor Project's on LGBTQ Youth Mental Health[15] is the largest survey thus far that represented over 40,000 LGBTQI youth, ages 13 to 24, across the United States.

[10] Ibid., para. 9-10.

[11] Bishop Joseph Strictland and Cardinal Raymond Burke, leaders of conservative Catholics in the United States views Francis's liberal stance towards homosexuality and approval of the blessing for homosexual couples in *Fiducia Supplicans* [Supplicating Trust] as a false blessing that can cause schism in the Church and undermining its moral teachings (Pierson 2023). Cardinal Gerhard Muller, the former head of the RCC's Congregation of the Doctrine of the Faith, saw Francis's approval of FS's liberal stance to homosexuality and blessing of gay couples by priests as blasphemous (Muller 2023), while the recently excommunicated Archbishop Carlo Maria Vigano (2023) characterized it as heresy.

---

15.   https://www.thetrevorproject.org/survey-2020/

Don't miss out!

Visit the website below and you can sign up to receive emails whenever Vivencio Ballano publishes a new book. There's no charge and no obligation.

https://books2read.com/r/B-A-ELMKC-KJOBF

BOOKS 2 READ

Connecting independent readers to independent writers.

Also by Vivencio Ballano

Gender and the Catholic Church
Why Can't Pope Francis and the Catholic Church Fully Accept the LGBTQI?:
A Sociological-Synodal Exploration and Solution
"We are God's Children Too!": Resisting Homophobia and Natural Law for Full
LGBTQI Integration in the Catholic Church
"We're Not an Ideology But Persons With Human Dignity"
Is Gender the Greatest Threat to Humanity and the Family?: A Sociological
Unmasking of a Moral Panic

My Religious Vocation and Journey Vol. 1
God's Call: Why I Entered the Seminary

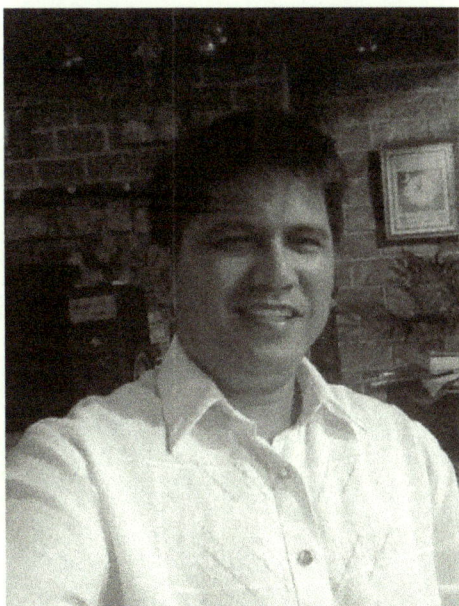

About the Author

Dr. Vivencio "Ven" Ballano holds a master's degree in Catholic theology and a doctorate in sociology from the Jesuit-run Ateneo de Manila University, Manila, Philippines. He is currently the Program Chairperson of the master's degree program in sociology at the Polytechnic University of the Philippines (PUP). To date, Dr. Ballano has published 7 Scopus-indexed books and 3 more forthcoming ones in 2024 and 2025 with imprints Springer Nature and Routledge.

Read more at https://www.researchgate.net/profile/Vivencio-Ballano/stats.

Milton Keynes UK
Ingram Content Group UK Ltd.
UKHW020021061124
450708UK00001B/285

9 798227 923479